The Quick & Easy DASH Diet Cookbook

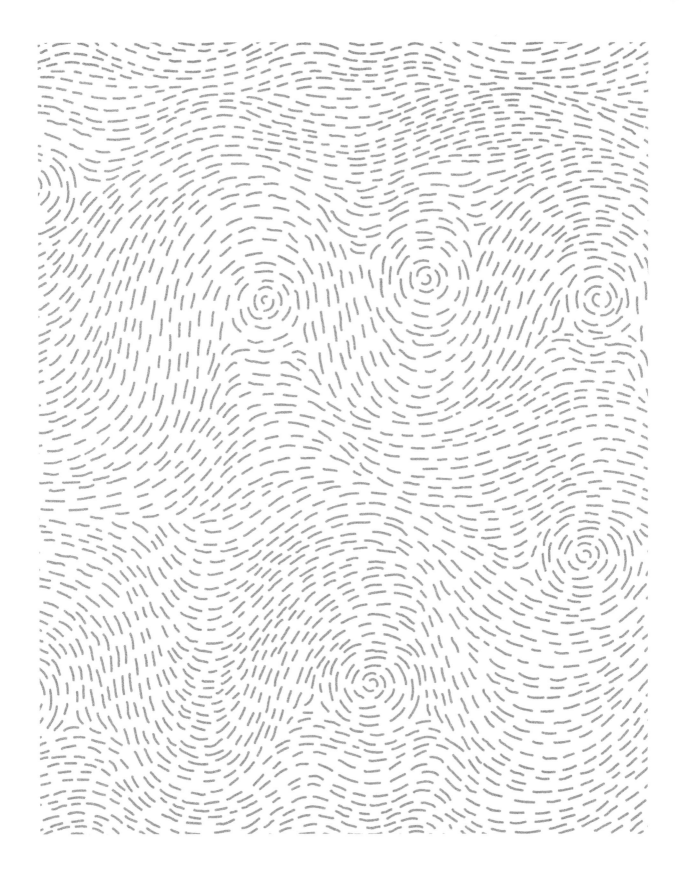

The Quick & Easy DASH Diet Cookbook

77 DASH DIET RECIPES
MADE IN MINUTES

ROCKRIDGE
PRESS

For general information on our other products and services or to obtain technical support, please contact our Customer Care Department within the United States at (866) 744-2665, or outside the United States at (510) 253-0500.

Rockridge Press publishes its books in a variety of electronic and print formats. Some content that appears in print may not be available in electronic books, and vice versa.

TRADEMARKS: Rockridge Press and the Rockridge Press logo are trademarks or registered trademarks of Callisto Media Inc. and/or its affiliates, in the United States and other countries, and may not be used without written permission. All other trademarks are the property of their respective owners. Rockridge Press is not associated with any product or vendor mentioned in this book.

ISBN: Print 978-1-62315-383-0 | eBook 978-1-62315-384-7

Table of Contents

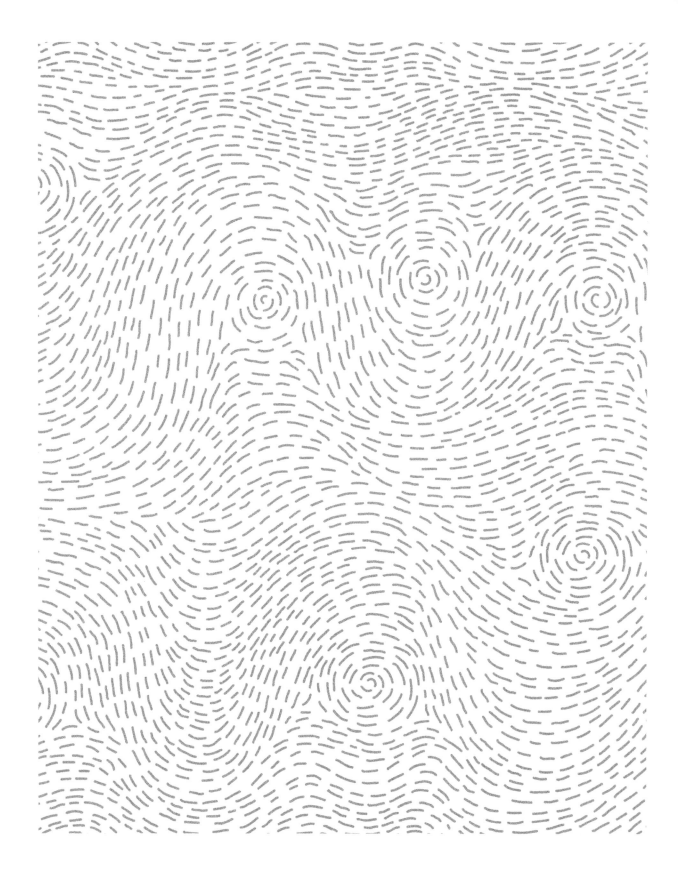

Introduction

Welcome to *The Quick & Easy DASH Diet Cookbook*. It's likely that you've picked up this book because you suffer from hypertension or are at risk for developing it. *DASH* stands for Dietary Approaches to Stop Hypertension, and the diet was created specifically to treat or prevent high blood pressure. While it is a very effective way to reduce blood pressure, the diet is also effective for weight loss as well as lowering cholesterol and helping prevent numerous diseases, including several types of cancer, heart disease, stroke, heart failure, kidney disease, type 2 diabetes, metabolic syndrome, and polycystic ovarian syndrome (PCOS).

As you'd expect, the diet encourages low-sodium eating, as well as limiting overall fat and saturated fat, sugar, and other caloric sweeteners. It includes a wide variety of foods that are rich in potassium, calcium, and magnesium, which help to lower blood pressure. It emphasizes eating a wide variety of health foods, including fruits and vegetables, low-fat dairy products, whole grains, and lean proteins.

The Quick & Easy DASH Diet Cookbook is filled with information that will help you incorporate the DASH diet into your life with ease. In addition to explaining the diet in accessible language and offering advice for incorporating the principles of the diet into your life, it also provides 77 quick and easy recipes that comply with the DASH diet guidelines. These recipes can be prepared in 30 minutes or less, using easy-to-find, affordable ingredients and standard kitchen equipment.

The book is divided into two parts. Part One explains what you need to know before getting started, including a detailed guide to kicking off your DASH diet. It examines the science behind the diet and the health benefits it offers. It includes lists of foods to eat and foods to avoid, and provides advice on meal planning, stocking your pantry, and cooking quick and delicious meals that adhere to the plan.

Part Two offers 77 quick and easy recipes that follow DASH diet guidelines. These dishes are a cinch to make, highly nutritious, and full of flavor. With these recipes in hand, you'll begin your DASH diet by eating delicious and satisfying meals. Since you'll be eating a wide variety of real foods, you'll find it easy to follow the plan and stick to it long-term.

By reading this book, you'll learn:

- Simple ways to incorporate the DASH diet into your daily life
- How to shop for DASH-friendly foods
- What foods contain health-enhancing vitamins, minerals, and other nutrients
- How to cook your favorite dishes with less sodium
- Delicious ways to add more fruits, vegetables, fiber, and lean protein to your meals

Remember that even small changes can have a quick and significant effect on your health. You may even find that your blood pressure drops in just a few weeks on the plan. Plus, more than likely, you'll lose weight, improve your overall health, and feel better than ever.

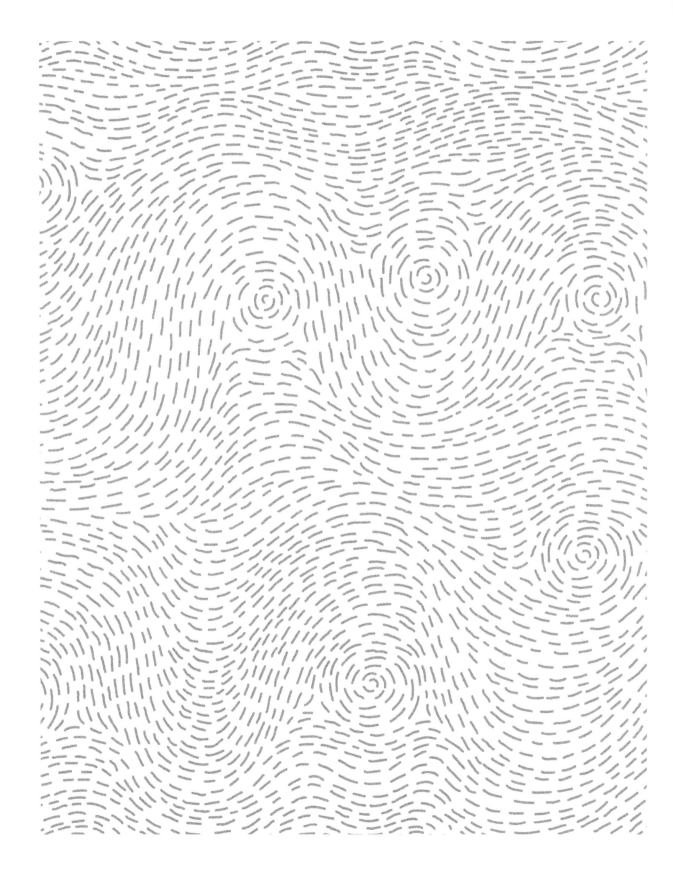

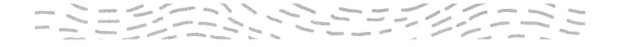

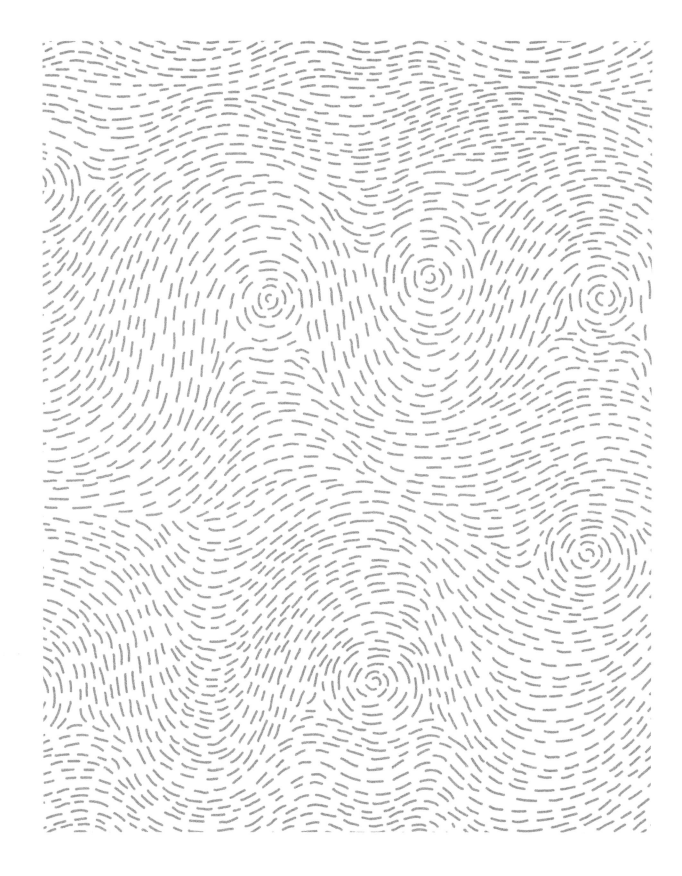

CHAPTER ONE

The Basics of the DASH Diet

The DASH diet is not just another fad diet. In fact, it is a lifetime eating strategy that the National Institutes of Health (NIH) developed through extensive research, in cooperation with five of the most highly respected medical research centers in the United States: Johns Hopkins University, Duke University Medical Center, Kaiser Permanente Center for Health Research, Brigham and Women's Hospital, and Pennington Biomedical Research Center.

The primary goal of the diet is to treat or prevent hypertension, but it has been shown to be a safe, healthy, easy-to-follow, and effective eating plan that helps fight numerous diseases and helps people lose weight. The diet emphasizes healthy eating strategies such as controlling portions and including lots of fresh fruits and vegetables, lean protein, and whole grains in meals.

WHAT IS THE DASH DIET?

The DASH diet was designed primarily to address the problem of hypertension. It is an eating plan that is low in sodium; it recommends a maximum daily sodium intake of 2,300 milligrams on the standard DASH diet and no more than 1,500 milligrams on the lower-sodium DASH diet. The latter is recommended for anyone who is over the age of 51 or African-American, or who suffers from hypertension, diabetes, or chronic kidney disease.

The diet is also high in fiber, lean protein, and minerals known to help reduce blood pressure, including potassium, calcium, and magnesium. It encourages strictly limiting portion sizes, overall fat and saturated fat, sweets, and caloric sweeteners.

People on the DASH diet eat lots of fresh fruits and vegetables, and moderate amounts of whole grains, low-fat and nonfat dairy, poultry, fish, meat, nuts, seeds, and beans. Sodium, added fats, red meat, high-fat dairy products, and added sugar are strictly limited.

BENEFITS OF THE DASH DIET

The connection between hypertension—which is believed to affect about fifty million people in the United States and as many as one billion worldwide—and the risk of cardiovascular disease is well documented. The higher your blood pressure, the greater your risk of heart attack, heart failure, stroke, and kidney disease. The DASH diet was developed specifically to provide those with hypertension a tool to get their condition under control in a way that would be easy to incorporate into their daily lives.

In studies sponsored by NIH, the DASH diet plan has been proved to lower blood pressure. Not a short-term diet, DASH is a healthy lifetime eating plan that is rich in fruits, vegetables, low-fat and nonfat dairy, lean proteins, and whole grains. It is designed to be low in sodium, high in fiber, low to moderate in fat, and rich in the blood-pressure-lowering minerals potassium, calcium, and magnesium.

At its core, the DASH diet is an eating plan that helps to lower blood pressure or prevent the onset of hypertension. And according to NIH research, it can significantly lower blood pressure in those who follow it.

Not just for those suffering from hypertension or at risk for developing it, the DASH diet is a sensible, well-balanced eating plan for anyone who wants to eat a healthy diet and reduce their risk of disease and/or lose weight.

WHAT TO EAT ON THE DASH DIET

A typical 2,000-calorie-per-day DASH daily meal plan looks like this:

- No more than 2,300 milligrams of sodium on the standard DASH diet or 1,500 milligrams on the lower-sodium DASH diet
- Six to eight servings of (ideally whole) grains (½ cup cooked pasta, rice, etc.; slice of bread; or 1 cup dry cereal per serving)
- Four to five servings of vegetables (1 cup raw leafy greens or ½ cup cooked vegetables per serving)
- Four to five servings of fruits (one medium fruit or ½ cup diced per serving)
- Two to three servings of low-fat or nonfat dairy (1 cup low-fat or nonfat milk or yogurt, 1 ounce reduced-fat cheese per serving)
- Up to six 1-ounce servings of fish, poultry, or lean meat
- Four to five 1½-ounce servings of nuts, seeds, and legumes
- Two to three servings of fats and oils (1 teaspoon oil or butter, 2 tablespoons salad dressing per serving)
- Up to one alcoholic beverage for women and up to two for men

Sweets should be strictly limited, with, at most, five servings per week of sweets (including low-fat desserts, fruit juices, and jams or jellies). Likewise, nuts, seeds, and legumes should be limited to about four to five servings per week.

One much-appreciated feature of the DASH diet is that it is an easy-to-follow eating plan that relies on common foods that are readily available in supermarkets and easy to prepare. There is no need to search out hard-to-find or expensive ingredients or tackle difficult cooking techniques. This plan relies on simple, whole foods to create delicious and satisfying meals.

Foods to Avoid

While the DASH diet doesn't strictly forbid any foods, the following should be avoided or eaten only in very small amounts.

- High-sodium foods, such as canned and prepared foods, salty snacks, most cheeses, and processed meats (hot dogs, sausages, salami, ham, etc.)
- High-fat and high-saturated-fat foods, like red meat and full-fat dairy products
- Foods containing trans fats
- Sugary beverages, including fruit juices and sodas

Foods to Enjoy

- Fruits—four to five servings per day
- Vegetables—four to five servings per day
- Whole grains and products made from whole grains—six to eight servings per day
- Fish, poultry, and lean meats—up to six servings per day
- Sweets, nuts, seeds, legumes, and alcohol in very limited quantities

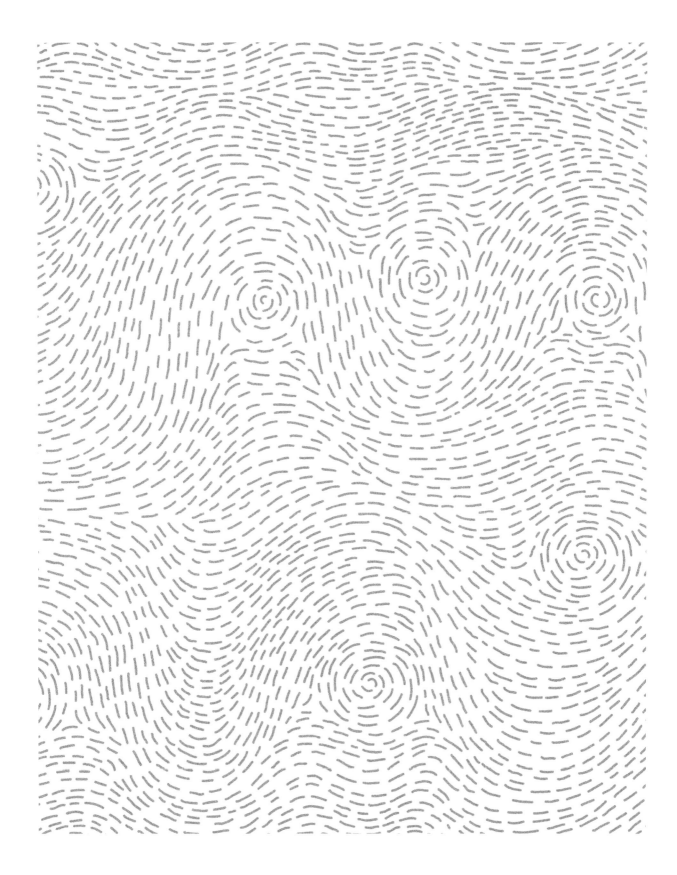

CHAPTER TWO

How to Save Time and Money

By now you understand what the DASH diet is and how it works to help you lower your blood pressure, lose weight, reduce your risk of disease, and improve your overall health. Now it's time to put the diet into action in your own life.

This chapter provides tips and advice for adopting the DASH diet quickly, easily, and without breaking the bank. You'll find suggestions on meal planning, stocking your pantry, grocery shopping, and cooking, so that a delicious DASH-friendly meal is always just minutes away.

PLAN AHEAD

As with any diet, meal plan, or lifestyle change, the biggest key to success is planning ahead. In order to make the change to the DASH way of eating, you'll need to stock up on certain DASH-friendly foods and rethink your day-to-day meal plan.

Create a Meal Plan

Read through the recipe section in this book, consult some other sources, and determine what you'll eat on each day of the upcoming week for breakfast, lunch, and dinner. Don't forget to think about snacks— both substantial snacks to serve as mini-meals as needed throughout the day, as well as those little nibbles that tide you over between meals. While it may seem time-consuming to write out a meal plan, it will ultimately save you time, not to mention money, to know exactly what you are going to eat and when. That way, you can make a shopping list that eliminates guesswork and makes it easy to buy everything you need in one shopping trip.

Don't put too much pressure on yourself. Not every meal has to be a gourmet feast. Many can be quick-cooking dishes you put together using simple ingredients, and any leftovers can become other meals. For instance, roast a chicken one night and serve it with roasted or steamed vegetables. The next day's breakfast can be scrambled eggs with leftover veggies. For lunch, have a salad with the leftover chicken.

MAKE A SHOPPING LIST

Once you have your meal plan ready to go, make a detailed shopping list that includes every ingredient for every dish or snack you plan to prepare, checking your pantry as you go to find out what you already have.

With your list in hand, you're much less likely to be tempted by enticing supermarket displays of off-limits foods. And by sticking to your list, you'll likely save time and money on your grocery shopping.

DASH Grocery Shopping Tips

- **Make a list and stick to it.**
  Make a list of everything you need for the week's meals and snacks, plus pantry items you need to replenish. Be sure to bring the list with you (or use a list-making app on your smart phone so you'll be sure to have it when you need it). Most important, don't allow yourself to be tempted by DASH unfriendly items. Stick to your list.
- **Buy fresh, whole foods whenever possible.**
  Processed or prepared foods often contain extremely high levels of sodium, not to mention added sugar and fat that you don't need or want in your diet. Fresh foods are a healthier choice because they generally contain less sodium, less fat, and no added sugar. By buying whole foods and preparing them yourself, you control exactly what and how much gets added to a meal before it hits your plate. Another advantage of fresh foods is that they are usually more nutritious—containing higher levels of vitamins, minerals, and fiber than processed foods—and more delicious.
- **Fill your cart with foods from the perimeter of the store first.**
  This is where the fresh produce, meats, fish, and dairy products are most often found. Venture into the center aisles only for specific DASH-friendly items such as whole-grain pasta, brown rice, whole-wheat bread, low-sodium broth, low-sodium canned beans, and low-sodium canned tomatoes.
- **Read the label every time.**
  Of course, you'll be buying mostly fresh foods that don't come with labels, but occasionally you'll want to use canned or processed foods for convenience. Be sure to read the labels carefully, choosing products that are low in sodium, added sugar, and saturated fat, and free of trans fats.
- **Never grocery shop on an empty stomach.**
  This is a recipe for disaster because hunger pangs can easily convince you to grab chips, cookies, or other unhealthy choices.

LEARN THE SIMPLE SKILLS FOR COOKING DASH-FRIENDLY MEALS

Eating prepared foods or eating out frequently makes following any healthy diet challenging, plus it's expensive. The best—and easiest—way to reduce the sodium, added sugar, and excess saturated fat in your diet, and save money at the same time, is to cook most of your food yourself. Then you know exactly what goes into it and can make your own adjustments—like adding spices to make up for less salt—guaranteeing that your food will be delicious. You'll even trim your food spending at the same time.

The more you cook healthful meals, the better you'll get at it. Seek out healthy recipes for your favorite foods, or adapt recipes yourself. Soon it will become second nature to substitute flavorful spices for added salt or switch out high-fat dairy for low-fat versions. Once you've mastered healthful cooking, almost no meal will be off limits to you. Whether it's pizza, tuna casserole, or spaghetti and meatballs you crave, you can adapt recipes to fit the DASH diet requirements.

Time- and Money-Saving Cooking Tips

- **Cook from scratch.**
  Preparing staples like beans and homemade broths from scratch, rather than turning to canned versions, will save you money. You control exactly what goes into your food, reducing the amount of added salt, sugar, and fat. If you cook large batches and freeze them in measured portions, using these homemade staples will be just as quick and easy as buying canned.

- **Watch your portion size.**
  A healthy serving of meat is just about 3 ounces (roughly the size of a deck of cards), but most people are accustomed to eating much more than that. Limit your portions to the sizes nutritionists recommend, especially for expensive and high-calorie foods such as meat and cheese, and you'll easily save money and cut your calorie intake. Instead, fill up your plate—and your belly—with low-calorie, highly nutritious, and inexpensive vegetables.

- **Roast large pieces of meat.**
  Roasting is a great way to cook meat without adding a lot of sodium or fat. Plus, roasted meats make great leftovers. Choose less expensive cuts, like turkey breast or pork shoulder, and you can eat for days for pennies per serving. Having leftovers to base additional meals on also saves you time in the kitchen.

- **Stir-fry your dinner.**
  Stir-frying is a quick cooking method that turns out flavorful and healthful one-pot meals. Load up your wok or skillet with lots of vegetables and just a little bit of meat for a meal that is quick, satisfying, nutritious, and inexpensive.

- **Prep once, cook twice.**
  When prepping commonly used foods—minced garlic, chopped onions, or diced celery—prep double (or triple) the amount you need and store the extra in a sealable bag in the fridge to use in a future recipe.

- **Double up for leftovers.**
  Double recipes for foods that keep well—soups, stews, casseroles, or roasted meats—so you have leftovers to eat for future meals. That way, you have saved time by only cooking once. It can also save you money, since it means you're more likely to use up perishable ingredients, like fresh herbs, that you bought specifically for a recipe.

- **Freeze it before you lose it.**

  Don't throw out overripe fruit. Dice it, pack it into freezer-safe plastic bags, and pop it in the freezer. Use it to sweeten smoothies, pancakes, muffins, or other foods.

- **Keep foods fresh.**

  Stock up on sealable, fridge- and freezer-safe containers for storing leftovers. Better still, invest in a vacuum sealer to ensure that frozen foods stay fresh and delicious for months.

- **Save time by cooking slow.**

  Investing in a slow cooker can save you lots of time in the kitchen. Toss ingredients into the cooker in the morning and come home to a complete meal of hearty vegetarian chili or vegetable-heavy meat stew. Pack up leftovers for future meals to save even more time, as well as money.

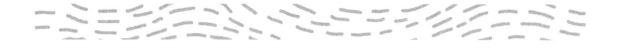

PART TWO

The Recipes

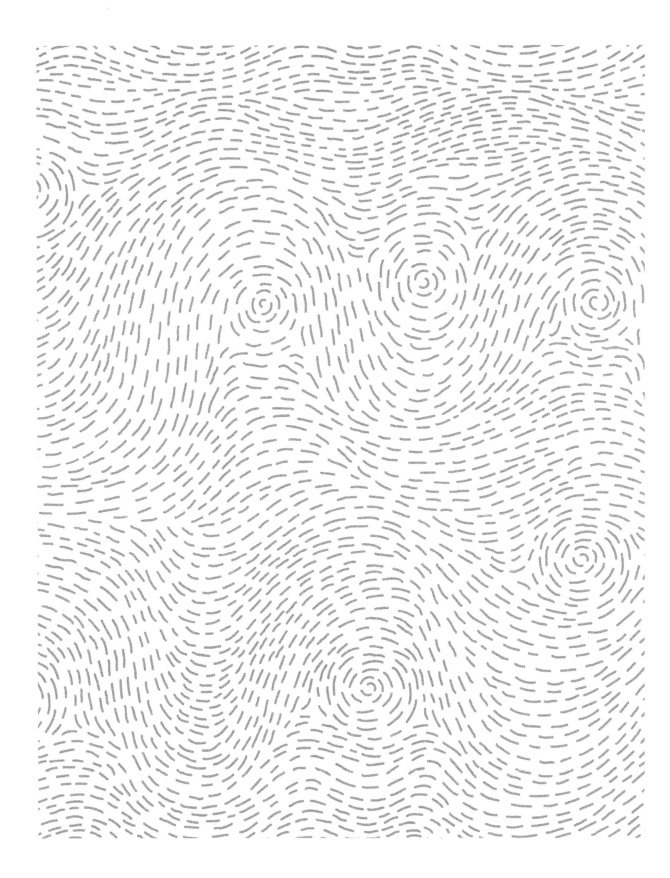

Breakfast

Banana–Peanut Butter Smoothie

SERVES 1

▶ CALORIES: **285**
    SODIUM: **186 MILLIGRAMS**

Prep time: **5 minutes**
Cooking time: **None**

This quick breakfast smoothie is low in sodium and loaded with blood-pressure-lowering potassium and calcium. For a thick smoothie that's cold and creamy like a milkshake, use a frozen banana (cut the banana into pieces before freezing).

1 CUP NONFAT MILK
1 TABLESPOON ALL-NATURAL CREAMY PEANUT BUTTER
1 BANANA

Combine the milk, peanut butter, and banana in a blender and process until smooth. Serve immediately.

Morning Muesli

SERVES 10

▶ CALORIES: **268**
  SODIUM: **48 MILLIGRAMS**

Prep time: **5 minutes**
Cooking time: **None**

Full of fruits, nuts, and heart-healthy oats, this delicious breakfast cereal is filling enough to keep you going until lunch. Mix up a large batch and keep it in an airtight container in your pantry for up to a month.

3 CUPS OLD FASHIONED ROLLED OATS
½ CUP NUTS (ALMONDS, MACADAMIAS, PECANS, WALNUTS, OR A COMBINATION)
½ CUP SESAME SEEDS
½ CUP SUNFLOWER SEEDS
½ CUP RAISINS
½ CUP DRIED, UNSWEETENED CRANBERRIES
1 CUP DRIED UNSWEETENED APRICOTS, CHOPPED

1. Combine all the ingredients in a large bowl.

2. To serve, add a cup of nonfat milk or yogurt, and fresh fruit. The dry muesli can be stored in an airtight container for up to one month.

Very Berry Breakfast Parfait

SERVES 4

▶ CALORIES: **237**
SODIUM: **88 MILLIGRAMS**

Prep time: **5 minutes**
Cooking time: **None**

Low in sodium, fat, and cholesterol, and packed with vitamin C and calcium, these gorgeous parfaits are a perfect start to the day. They're so pretty and flavorful, you could even serve them as a healthful dessert.

1½ CUPS PLAIN LOW-FAT YOGURT

3 TABLESPOONS HONEY

1½ CUPS MUESLI BREAKFAST CEREAL (SEE MORNING MUESLI, PAGE 17) OR LOW-SODIUM, LOW-FAT GRANOLA

1½ CUPS MIXED FRESH BERRIES (BLACKBERRIES, BLUEBERRIES, RASPBERRIES, OR SLICED STRAWBERRIES IN ANY COMBINATION)

1. In a small mixing bowl, combine the yogurt and honey, and stir to mix well.

2. Have four parfait glasses, 8-ounce mason jars, or other glasses ready. Spoon 2 tablespoons of the yogurt mixture into the bottom of each glass. Top with 2 tablespoons of the cereal, then 2 tablespoons of the fruit. Repeat until all of the ingredients have been used.

3. Serve immediately, or cover and refrigerate for up to 2 hours.

Creamy Strawberry Oatmeal

SERVES 1

▶ CALORIES: **313**
SODIUM: **77 MILLIGRAMS**

Prep time: **3 minutes**
Cooking time: **5 minutes**

Oatmeal is full of fiber, which keeps you feeling full. Fiber also reduces cholesterol and limits your risk for numerous diseases, including diabetes, high blood pressure, heart disease, and cancer. This version is creamy, sweet, and loaded with vitamin C. Feel free to substitute other fruits, such as bananas, peaches, or pears as the seasons change.

½ CUP WATER

¼ CUP LOW-FAT MILK

½ CUP OLD-FASHIONED ROLLED OATS

½ CUP SLICED STRAWBERRIES

¼ CUP NONFAT GREEK YOGURT

1 TABLESPOON HONEY

1. In a small saucepan set over medium heat, combine the water, milk, and oats. Bring the mixture to a boil, stirring occasionally.

2. Reduce the heat to low and simmer for 3 to 5 minutes, stirring occasionally, until the oats are tender. Remove from the heat, cover, and let stand for 3 to 5 minutes.

3. Transfer to a serving bowl. Stir in the strawberries, yogurt, and honey, and serve immediately.

Date-Sweetened Chocolate Oatmeal

SERVES 2

▶ CALORIES: **281**
   SODIUM: **61 MILLIGRAMS**

Prep time: **5 minutes**
Cooking time: **2 minutes**

What better way to start your day than with a bowl of nutritious oatmeal flavored with chocolate? It's even better for you when using dates for sweetness instead of refined sugar.

1 CUP LOW-FAT MILK
1 CUP WATER
1 CUP OLD-FASHIONED ROLLED OATS
¼ CUP CHOPPED PITTED DATES (10 TO 12 DATES)
2 TABLESPOONS UNSWEETENED COCOA

1. Combine all the ingredients in a medium saucepan set over medium heat and heat until almost boiling.

2. Cook, stirring constantly, for about 2 minutes, until the mixture is creamy. Serve hot.

Cinnamon-Apple Quinoa Breakfast Bowl

SERVES 6

▶ CALORIES: **239**
SODIUM: **9 MILLIGRAMS**

Prep time: **5 minutes**
Cooking time: **15 minutes**

Quinoa is popular among health-conscious eaters for a reason. It is rich in protein and a great source of fiber and magnesium, which help lower blood pressure and keep blood sugar stable. This dish is a great way to start your day.

1 CUP UNSWEETENED ALMOND MILK

1 CUP WATER

1 CUP UNCOOKED QUINOA

½ TEASPOON GROUND CINNAMON

½ APPLE, DICED SMALL

⅓ CUP CHOPPED PECANS

2 TABLESPOONS RAISINS

1. In a medium saucepan, combine the almond milk, water, quinoa, and cinnamon, and bring to a boil. Reduce the heat to medium-low and simmer until most of the liquid is absorbed, about 15 minutes.

2. Stir in the apple, pecans, and raisins and serve immediately.

Lemon-Blueberry Muffins

MAKES 12 MUFFINS

▶ CALORIES: **177**
SODIUM: **133 MILLIGRAMS**

Prep time: **5 minutes**
Cooking time: **25 minutes**

Low-fat buttermilk makes these quick muffins super moist and gives them a rich, tangy flavor. Make these muffins when antioxidant-rich blueberries are at their peak in summer, or anytime of year using frozen berries (they'll be just as delicious).

1 CUP WHITE WHOLE-WHEAT FLOUR

1 CUP ALL-PURPOSE FLOUR

2 TEASPOONS BAKING POWDER

1 TEASPOON BAKING SODA

⅓ CUP GRANULATED SUGAR

ZEST OF 1 LEMON, FINELY GRATED

1 CUP LOW-FAT BUTTERMILK

⅓ CUP CANOLA OIL

1 EGG

1 TEASPOON VANILLA EXTRACT

1½ CUPS FRESH OR FROZEN (NOT THAWED) BLUEBERRIES

1. Preheat the oven to 400°F. Line a standard 12-cup muffin tin with paper liners or spray with nonstick cooking spray.

2. In a medium mixing bowl, combine the whole-wheat and all-purpose flours, baking powder, and baking soda.

3. In a large mixing bowl, combine the sugar, lemon zest, buttermilk, canola oil, egg, and vanilla, and beat using an electric mixer on medium speed until well combined.

4. Add the dry ingredients to the wet ingredients in two or three batches, beating just to combine after each addition. Gently fold in the blueberries.

5. Spoon the batter evenly into the prepared muffin cups. Bake in the preheated oven for 20 to 25 minutes, until the tops are golden and a toothpick inserted into the center comes out clean.

6. Let the muffins cool in the pan for a few minutes, then transfer to a wire rack. Serve warm or at room temperature.

Maple-Cinnamon Oatmeal Pancakes

SERVES 4

▶   CALORIES: **259**
SODIUM: **150 MILLIGRAMS**

Prep time: **15 minutes** (includes standing time)
Cooking time: **15 minutes**

Low-fat buttermilk adds flavor and protein to these healthful fiber-rich pancakes. Serve them with fresh fruit, yogurt, powdered sugar, or additional maple syrup for drizzling.

1½ CUPS OLD-FASHIONED ROLLED OATS
½ CUP WHOLE-WHEAT FLOUR
1 TEASPOON GROUND CINNAMON
1 TEASPOON BAKING POWDER
2 CUPS LOW-FAT BUTTERMILK
2 TABLESPOONS MAPLE SYRUP
1 EGG
COOKING SPRAY

1. In a medium mixing bowl, combine the oats, flour, cinnamon, and baking powder.

2. In a large mixing bowl, whisk together the buttermilk, maple syrup, and egg.

3. Add the dry mixture to the wet mixture in two or three batches, mixing well after each addition. Let stand for about 10 minutes, until the mixture becomes bubbly.

4. Spray a nonstick skillet with cooking spray and heat over medium heat. For each pancake, use about ¼ cup batter, and cook for 2 to 3 minutes, until bubbles appear on the surface. Flip over and continue to cook for 1 to 2 minutes, until browned on the other side. Cook the remaining batter in batches of three or four until finished. Serve immediately.

No-Bake Peanut Butter Power Bars

SERVES 8

▶ CALORIES: **187** (PER BAR)
SODIUM: **2 MILLIGRAMS** (PER BAR)

Prep time: **30 minutes** (includes chilling time)
Cooking time: **None**

Peanut butter has a magic combination of fiber and protein that fills you up and keeps you feeling full. It also delivers a big dose of blood-pressure-lowering potassium. These nutrition-packed bars are quick to make and great to have around for those days when you have no time to make breakfast.

1¾ CUPS PITTED DATES
½ CUP UNSWEETENED DRIED CRANBERRIES
¼ CUP ALL-NATURAL PEANUT BUTTER
¼ CUP WHOLE RAW ALMONDS
½ CUP INSTANT OATS

1. Place the dates in a small bowl and cover with warm water. Let sit for 10 minutes, then drain.

2. In a food processor, combine the dates, cranberries, peanut butter, almonds, and oats, and process to a paste.

3. Press the mixture into an 8-by-8-inch nonstick baking pan in an even layer.

4. Chill in the freezer for 15 minutes to set. Cut into bars and serve immediately, or store in the fridge for up to 2 weeks or in the freezer for up to 3 months.

Spiced Whole-Grain Zucchini Pancakes

SERVES 4

▶ CALORIES: **291**
  SODIUM: **116 MILLIGRAMS**

Prep time: **10 minutes**
Cooking time: **15 minutes**

Get your veggie servings in early with these zucchini-packed pancakes that taste like pumpkin pie. Serve them topped with yogurt, fresh fruit, or maple syrup.

2 CUPS SHREDDED ZUCCHINI
1¼ CUPS WHOLE-WHEAT FLOUR
2 TEASPOONS BAKING POWDER
1 TEASPOON PUMPKIN PIE SPICE
2 EGGS
1 CUP PLUS 2 TABLESPOONS LOW-FAT MILK
2 TABLESPOONS UNSALTED BUTTER, MELTED
2 TABLESPOONS LIGHT BROWN SUGAR
1 TEASPOON VANILLA EXTRACT
COOKING SPRAY

1. Wrap the shredded zucchini in a clean dish towel and squeeze out as much water as possible.

2. In a large bowl, combine the flour, baking powder, and pumpkin pie spice.

3. In a medium bowl, whisk together the eggs, milk, butter, brown sugar, and vanilla. Add the wet ingredients to the dry ingredients and whisk to combine. Stir in the zucchini.

4. Spray a large nonstick skillet with cooking spray and heat over medium heat. For each pancake, use about ⅓ cup batter (about 4 inches in diameter) and cook for 2 to 3 minutes, until bubbles appear on the surface. If the batter is too thick, add a splash of milk. Flip the pancakes over and cook 1 to 2 minutes, until the other side is golden brown. Serve hot.

Mini Frittata Muffins

SERVES 8

▶ CALORIES: **47**
   SODIUM: **143 MILLIGRAMS**

Prep time: **10 minutes**
Cooking time: **20 minutes**

These frittatas make a great on-the-go breakfast. Full of protein, they'll fill you up and get your day started right.

COOKING SPRAY
½ ONION, FINELY DICED
⅔ CUP (ABOUT 2 OUNCES) CHOPPED REDUCED-FAT HAM
4 EGG WHITES
1 EGG
⅓ CUP (ABOUT 1½ OUNCES) SHREDDED REDUCED-FAT EXTRA-SHARP CHEDDAR CHEESE
2 TABLESPOONS CHOPPED FRESH CHIVES
⅛ TEASPOON FRESHLY GROUND PEPPER

1. Preheat the oven to 350°F. Spray a 24-cup mini muffin tin with cooking spray.

2. Spray a large nonstick skillet with cooking spray and heat over medium-high heat. Add the onion and cook, stirring, just until it begins to soften, about 2 minutes. Add the ham and cook, stirring, for 2 minutes, until it is crisp-tender.

3. In a large bowl, whisk together the egg whites, egg, cheese, chives, and pepper. Stir in the ham-onion mixture.

4. Spoon the egg mixture into the prepared muffin tin and bake in the preheated oven until set, about 20 minutes.

5. Serve warm or at room temperature. The muffins can be stored in the refrigerator for up to a week or in the freezer for up to a month. Reheat in a microwave or set on the counter and allow them to come to room temperature before serving.

Spicy Baked Eggs with Goat Cheese and Spinach

SERVES 4

▶ CALORIES: **156**
  SODIUM: **272 MILLIGRAMS**

Prep time: **5 minutes**
Cooking time: **20 minutes**

Baking eggs in a muffin tin or in ramekins is an easy way to cook eggs for several people at once. This version combines iron-rich spinach, spicy salsa for a little kick, and naturally low-fat goat cheese for richness and tang.

COOKING SPRAY
10 OUNCES FROZEN CHOPPED SPINACH, THAWED AND SQUEEZED DRY
4 EGGS
¼ CUP CHUNKY SALSA
¼ CUP CRUMBLED GOAT CHEESE
FRESHLY GROUND PEPPER TO TASTE

1. Preheat the oven to 325°F. Spray four 6-ounce ramekins with cooking spray.

2. For each ramekin, cover the bottom with spinach. Make a slight indentation in the center of the spinach and crack an egg into it. Top the egg with 1 tablespoon of the salsa and 1 tablespoon of the goat cheese. Sprinkle with pepper.

3. Place the ramekins on a baking sheet and bake in the preheated oven for about 20 minutes, until the whites are completely set but the yolk is still a bit runny. Serve immediately.

Super-Fast Breakfast Burrito

SERVES 4

▶ CALORIES: **354**
SODIUM: **402 MILLIGRAMS**

Prep time: **5 minutes**
Cooking time: **5 minutes**

Making eggs in the microwave is a quick, mess-free way to get a healthy breakfast on the table in just minutes. Black beans add extra fiber and protein to this flavorful breakfast wrap.

4 EGG WHITES
2 EGGS
¼ CUP LOW-FAT MILK
⅛ TEASPOON FRESHLY GROUND PEPPER
4 WHOLE-WHEAT TORTILLAS
½ CUP (2 OUNCES) SHREDDED REDUCED-FAT SHARP CHEDDAR CHEESE
1 CUP CANNED BLACK BEANS, RINSED AND DRAINED
¼ CUP CHOPPED SCALLIONS
½ CUP SALSA
¼ CUP NONFAT SOUR CREAM

1. In a microwave-safe dish, whisk together the egg whites, eggs, milk, and pepper. Cook the mixture in the microwave on high for 3 minutes. Remove the dish from the microwave and stir. Microwave for 1 additional minute, or until the eggs are set.

2. Arrange 1 tortilla on each of four microwave-safe plates. Divide the egg mixture evenly over the tortillas. Top each with one quarter of the cheese, beans, and scallions.

3. Wrap the burritos up and microwave for 30 seconds. Serve immediately, topped with salsa and sour cream.

Poached Eggs and Asparagus on Toast

SERVES 4

▶ CALORIES: **301**
   SODIUM: **323 MILLIGRAMS**

Prep time: **5 minutes**
Cooking time: **15 minutes**

Asparagus somehow makes any meal seem like a special occasion. Celebrate the morning with this simple yet satisfying breakfast.

4 SLICES WHOLE-WHEAT SOURDOUGH BREAD
1 POUND ASPARAGUS, TRIMMED
2 TABLESPOONS OLIVE OIL
½ TEASPOON FRESHLY GROUND PEPPER
8 EGGS
¼ CUP (ABOUT 1 OUNCE) GRATED PARMESAN CHEESE

1. Preheat the broiler. Set a saucepan of water over medium-high heat and bring to a boil.

2. Arrange the bread and asparagus on a large rimmed baking sheet, drizzle with the olive oil, and sprinkle with the pepper. Broil in the preheated oven for about 1 to 2 minutes, until the bread is toasted on top. Flip the bread over and broil for 1 to 2 minutes more, until the other side is toasted. Transfer the bread to four serving plates and return the asparagus to the broiler. Broil for 5 to 8 minutes, until tender.

3. Meanwhile, with the water in the saucepan at a simmer, carefully crack the eggs into it. Reduce the heat to medium-low and simmer for about 4 minutes, until the whites are set and the yolks are still runny.

4. Arrange the asparagus equally over the toast. Top each slice with 2 eggs and sprinkle with the cheese. Serve immediately.

Sweet Potato Hash with Brussels Sprouts and Soft-Boiled Eggs

SERVES 4

▶ CALORIES: **245**
SODIUM: **83 MILLIGRAMS**

Prep time: **5 minutes**
Cooking time: **20 minutes**

Orange-fleshed sweet potatoes, which are full of beta-carotene and fiber, are much more nutritious than their white-potato counterparts. Here, they're combined with Brussels sprouts and red onions and topped with soft-boiled eggs.

2 TABLESPOONS OLIVE OIL

2 GARLIC CLOVES, MINCED

½ RED ONION, DICED

2 SWEET POTATOES, PEELED AND DICED

8 OUNCES BRUSSELS SPROUTS, TRIMMED AND SLICED CROSSWISE

1 TEASPOON MINCED FRESH THYME

½ TEASPOON FRESHLY GROUND PEPPER

4 EGGS

1. Fill a medium saucepan with about 4 inches of water and bring to a boil over high heat.

2. Meanwhile, heat the olive oil in a large skillet over medium heat. Add the garlic and cook, stirring, for 1 minute. Add the onion and cook, stirring occasionally, until it begins to soften, about 2 to 3 minutes.

3. Increase the heat to medium-high and add the sweet potatoes. Cook, stirring occasionally, until the potatoes begin to brown, about 8 minutes. Add the Brussels sprouts and cook for 4 or 5 minutes, until they begin to brown. Season with thyme and pepper.

4. When the water in the saucepan is boiling, carefully add the eggs. Reduce the heat to low and simmer for 6 minutes. Drain and rinse the eggs under cold water.

5. Divide the hash evenly among four serving plates. Carefully peel the eggs and place one on top of each serving of hash. Serve immediately.

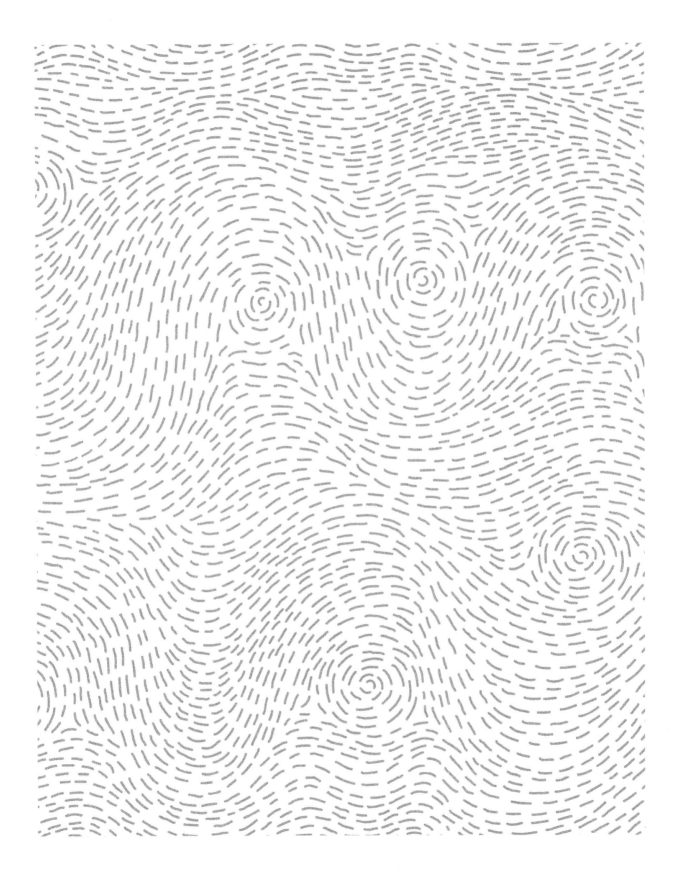

CHAPTER FOUR

Snacks and Appetizers

Roasted Plums with Greek Yogurt

SERVES 4

▶ CALORIES: **111**
   SODIUM: **16 MILLIGRAMS**

Prep time: **3 minutes**
Cooking time: **15 minutes**

Roasting fruit intensifies its sweetness and brings out a caramelized flavor. These roasted plums are paired with a dollop of yogurt and a sprinkling of hazelnuts for a midday snack.

6 PLUMS, HALVED AND PITTED
COOKING SPRAY
2 TEASPOONS GRANULATED SUGAR
½ CUP LOW-FAT GREEK YOGURT
2 TABLESPOONS CHOPPED TOASTED HAZELNUTS
2 TEASPOONS HONEY

1. Preheat the oven to 375°F. Line a baking sheet with parchment paper.

2. Arrange the plums cut-side up on the baking sheet, spray with cooking spray, and sprinkle with sugar. Bake the plums in the preheated oven until they begin to soften and brown a bit, about 15 minutes.

3. Divide the plums evenly among four serving bowls and top each with a dollop of yogurt, a sprinkle of nuts, and a drizzle of honey. Serve immediately.

Spicy Popcorn

SERVES 4

▶ CALORIES: **115**
SODIUM: **64 MILLIGRAMS**

Prep time: **2 minutes**
Cooking time: **None**

Popcorn is a whole grain, but the movie theater version—popped in oil, drenched in butter, and heavily salted—is a DASH diet no-no. This spicy version lets you enjoy popcorn's whole-grain goodness without a hint of guilt.

½ TEASPOON CHILI POWDER

⅛ TEASPOON SALT-FREE GARLIC POWDER

⅛ TEASPOON PAPRIKA

⅛ TEASPOON CAYENNE

8 CUPS AIR-POPPED POPCORN

1. In a small bowl, combine the chili powder, garlic powder, paprika, and cayenne.

2. Place the popcorn in a large bowl and toss with the spice mixture. Serve immediately or store in an airtight container for up to 2 days.

Baked Spiced Tortilla Chips

SERVES 6

▶   CALORIES: **127**
SODIUM: **23 MILLIGRAMS**

Prep time: **5 minutes**
Cooking time: **25 minutes**

Sometimes you just need something crunchy to scoop up salsa and guacamole with. These flavorful baked tortilla chips do the trick.

COOKING SPRAY
4 TEASPOONS LIME JUICE
2 TEASPOONS CANOLA OIL
½ TEASPOON GROUND CUMIN
12 SIX-INCH CORN TORTILLAS

1. Preheat the oven to 400°F. Spray two large baking sheets with cooking spray.

2. In a small bowl, stir together the lime juice, canola oil, and cumin. Brush each tortilla on both sides with the mixture and cut each into 6 wedges.

3. Arrange the tortilla pieces in a single layer on the prepared baking sheets. Bake in the preheated oven, rotating the pans every 10 minutes, until the chips are golden brown and crisp, about 25 minutes.

Pumpkin Seed Party Mix

SERVES 6

▶ CALORIES: **114**
SODIUM: **119 MILLIGRAMS**

Prep time: **5 minutes**
Cooking time: **20 minutes**

Pumpkin seeds are loaded with blood-pressure-lowering magnesium, as well as immune-system-boosting zinc and omega-3 fatty acids. This crunchy, spicy party mix is addictive, but it's an addiction that will improve your health rather than compromise it.

COOKING SPRAY

2 CUPS CRISPY RICE CEREAL SQUARES (SUCH AS RICE CHEX)

½ CUP UNSALTED ROASTED PUMPKIN SEEDS

⅓ CUP SLIVERED ALMONDS

1 TABLESPOON CANOLA OIL

2 TEASPOONS CHILI POWDER

2 TEASPOONS WORCESTERSHIRE SAUCE

2 TEASPOONS PREPARED MUSTARD

½ TEASPOON SMOKED PAPRIKA

¼ TEASPOON GROUND CUMIN

¼ TEASPOON CAYENNE

1. Preheat the oven to 300°F. Spray a large rimmed baking sheet with cooking spray.

2. In a large bowl, combine the rice cereal, pumpkin seeds, and almonds.

3. In a small bowl, stir together the canola oil, chili powder, Worcestershire sauce, mustard, paprika, cumin, and cayenne. Drizzle the mixture over the cereal mixture and toss to coat well.

4. Spread the cereal mixture out in a single layer on the prepared baking sheet and bake in the preheated oven for about 20 minutes, stirring once halfway through the baking, until the mixture begins to brown and becomes crisp. Transfer the pan to a wire rack to cool.

5. Serve at room temperature. The party mix can be stored in an airtight container on the countertop for up to a week.

Hard-Boiled Eggs with Paprika Oil

SERVES 4

▶ CALORIES: **94**
   SODIUM: **62 MILLIGRAMS**

Prep time: **12 minutes** (includes standing time)
Cooking time: **1 minute**

Bright orange paprika oil brings simple hard-boiled eggs to life. Serve this high-protein canapé as a simple party appetizer or first course, or just eat it as a midday snack.

1 TABLESPOON OLIVE OIL
½ TEASPOON PAPRIKA
4 HARD-BOILED EGGS, CUT IN HALF
1 TABLESPOON MINCED FLAT-LEAF PARSLEY

1. Place the olive oil in a small, microwave-safe dipping bowl and heat in the microwave in 30-second intervals until hot. Stir in the paprika and let sit for 10 minutes.

2. Arrange the egg slices on a platter, drizzle with the oil, and sprinkle with the parsley. Serve immediately.

Bruschetta

▶ CALORIES: **120**
  SODIUM: **172 MILLIGRAMS**

Prep time: **25 minutes** (includes standing time)
Cooking time: **None**

The simple flavors of fresh tomatoes, garlic, and fresh basil make this a heavenly appetizer. Tomatoes are loaded with vitamin C, and garlic is a disease-fighting nutritional wonder.

4 PLUM TOMATOES, CHOPPED
¼ CUP MINCED FRESH BASIL
2 TEASPOONS OLIVE OIL
1 GARLIC CLOVE, MINCED
4 OUNCES CRUSTY ITALIAN PEASANT BREAD, CUT INTO 4 SLICES AND TOASTED
FRESHLY GROUND PEPPER TO TASTE

1. In a medium bowl, stir together the tomatoes, basil, olive oil, and garlic. Cover and let stand for 20 minutes to blend the flavors.

2. Divide the tomato mixture evenly over the toasted bread and drizzle any remaining juice over the top. Sprinkle with pepper and serve immediately.

Zucchini-Parmesan Chips

SERVES 4

▶ CALORIES: **70**
SODIUM: **128 MILLIGRAMS**

Prep time: **5 minutes**
Cooking time: **20 minutes**

These crispy, golden brown zucchini rounds are much more healthful than traditional deep-fried zucchini, but no less delicious. A little bit of Parmesan adds a lot of flavor.

COOKING SPRAY
¼ CUP DRY BREAD CRUMBS
¼ CUP (1 OUNCE) GRATED PARMESAN CHEESE
¼ TEASPOON SALT-FREE GARLIC POWDER
⅛ TEASPOON FRESHLY GROUND PEPPER
2 TABLESPOONS NONFAT MILK
2 ZUCCHINI, SLICED INTO ¼-INCH-THICK ROUNDS

1. Preheat the oven to 450°F. Place an oven-safe wire rack on a large baking sheet and spray it with cooking spray.

2. In a medium bowl, whisk together the bread crumbs, cheese, garlic powder, and pepper.

3. Put the milk in a shallow bowl.

4. Dip the zucchini slices first in the milk and then in the bread-crumb mixture, making sure to coat the zucchini well. Arrange the zucchini slices on the prepared rack and bake in the preheated oven until golden brown and crisp, about 20 minutes. Serve immediately.

Chipotle Guacamole

SERVES 4

▶ CALORIES: **105**
SODIUM: **5 MILLIGRAMS**

Prep time: **5 minutes**
Cooking time: **None**

Avocados are full of healthy fats that help prevent cardiovascular disease and diabetes while supporting weight maintenance and nutrient absorption. Serve with Baked Spiced Tortilla Chips (page 36) for a healthy and delicious party snack.

1 AVOCADO
1 TOMATO, SEEDED AND DICED
1½ TABLESPOONS FINELY DICED RED ONION
1 TABLESPOON LIME JUICE
1 TABLESPOON MINCED CILANTRO
⅛ TO ¼ TEASPOON GROUND CHIPOTLE

1. Halve the avocado, remove the pit, and use a large spoon to scoop out the flesh into a medium bowl. Mash the avocado with a fork, leaving it a bit lumpy.

2. Add the tomato, onion, lime juice, cilantro, and chipotle and stir to mix well. Serve immediately.

Roasted Red Pepper Hummus

SERVES 6

▶ CALORIES: **317**
   SODIUM: **72 MILLIGRAMS**

Prep time: **5 minutes**
Cooking time: **None**

Store-bought hummus, while full of protein, fiber, vitamins, and minerals, is usually sodium-heavy. This homemade version is quick to make and relies on roasted peppers and spices, not salt, for flavor. Serve this tasty dip with crudités or whole-wheat pita triangles for a healthy snack or appetizer.

ONE 15-OUNCE CAN CHICKPEAS

½ CUP JARRED ROASTED RED BELL PEPPERS, DRAINED

1 GARLIC CLOVE

¼ CUP LEMON JUICE

2 TABLESPOONS TAHINI (SESAME PASTE)

1 TABLESPOON OLIVE OIL

¼ TEASPOON GROUND CUMIN

⅛ TEASPOON CAYENNE

1. Process the chickpeas, red peppers, and garlic in a food processor until smooth.

2. Add the lemon juice, tahini, olive oil, cumin, and cayenne, and process to blend well. If the mixture is too thick, add water, 1 tablespoon at a time, until it reaches the desired consistency. Serve immediately or cover and refrigerate for up to 2 days.

Fresh Garlic and Herb Yogurt Dip

SERVES 8

▶ CALORIES: **62**
   SODIUM: **16 MILLIGRAMS**

Prep time: **25 minutes** (includes standing time)
Cooking time: **None**

Who doesn't love a creamy onion dip with crispy potato chips? This yogurt-based version is loaded with herbs and fresh garlic, keeping it healthy, light, and delicious. Serve it with baked potato chips or fresh vegetable crudités for a satisfying snack.

1 CUP NONFAT GREEK YOGURT

½ CUP GRATED CUCUMBER, DRAINED AND SQUEEZED DRY

2 TABLESPOONS GRATED YELLOW ONION

1 TABLESPOON MINCED FRESH DILL

1 TABLESPOON LEMON JUICE

1 TABLESPOON MINCED FRESH MINT

1 TEASPOON MINCED FRESH OREGANO

2 TEASPOONS HONEY

2 GARLIC CLOVES, MINCED

1 TEASPOON OLIVE OIL

1. In a medium bowl, combine all the ingredients and stir together until well combined. Let stand for 20 minutes to blend the flavors.

2. Serve immediately, or store, covered, in the refrigerator for up to 2 days.

Wasabi and Cream Cheese–Filled Snow Peas

SERVES 6

▶ CALORIES: **116**
  SODIUM: **61 MILLIGRAMS**

Prep time: **10 minutes**
Cooking time: **1 minute**

These adorable canapés make a good everyday snack or a healthy offering at your next party.
Adjust the amount of wasabi paste to suit your taste.

24 SNOW PEAS, STRINGS REMOVED
½ CUP LOW-FAT WHIPPED CREAM CHEESE
2 OR 3 TABLESPOONS WASABI PASTE
½ TEASPOON FRESHLY GROUND PEPPER
4 OR 5 RADISHES, THINLY SLICED
1 TABLESPOON SESAME SEEDS

1. Gently break open the top edge of each of the snow peas without splitting it apart. Arrange the snow peas on a serving platter.

2. In a small bowl, stir together the cream cheese, wasabi paste, and pepper until well combined. Transfer the mixture to a heavy-duty resealable plastic bag. Snip off a corner of the bag and pipe the cream cheese mixture into the snow peas.

3. Insert 2 or 3 radish slices into the cream cheese in each snow pea.

4. Heat a cast-iron or heavy skillet over high heat and toast the sesame seeds, shaking constantly, for about 1 minute, until toasted. Remove them from the skillet, let cool, and sprinkle them over the filled snow peas. Serve immediately.

Curried Zucchini and Goat Cheese Rolls

SERVES 6

▶   CALORIES: **87**
    SODIUM: **57 MILLIGRAMS**

Prep time: **5 minutes**
Cooking time: **10 minutes**

Tangy goat cheese is naturally low-fat. Here it's used to hold together spicy curry-roasted zucchini in pretty, party-worthy roll-ups.

4½ TEASPOONS CURRY POWDER
½ TEASPOON SALT-FREE GARLIC POWDER
⅛ TEASPOON CAYENNE
2 ZUCCHINI, SLICED LENGTHWISE INTO ⅛-INCH-THICK SLICES
COOKING SPRAY
1 JAR ROASTED RED BELL PEPPERS, DRAINED, RINSED, AND CUT INTO THIN STRIPS
3 OUNCES GOAT CHEESE

1. In a small bowl, combine the curry powder, garlic powder, and cayenne.

2. Spray the zucchini slices on both sides with the cooking spray. Rub the spice mixture on both sides of the zucchini.

3. Preheat a grill pan or outdoor grill to high heat. Grill the zucchini in a single layer until they are golden brown and slightly charred, about 4 to 5 minutes per side.

4. Crumble goat cheese down the length of each zucchini strip and top each with a roasted pepper strip. Roll the slices up and arrange on a serving platter, seam-side down. Serve chilled or at room temperature.

Crispy Salmon Cakes with Creamy Sun-Dried Tomato and Garlic Sauce

SERVES 8

▶ CALORIES: **154**
SODIUM: **109 MILLIGRAMS**

Prep time: **5 minutes**
Cooking time: **20 minutes**

Full of omega-3 fatty acids, salmon is a darling of the nutrition world. These salmon cakes let you reap the benefits of this healthy fish with little effort and lots of flavor.

SAUCE

¼ CUP SUN-DRIED TOMATOES (DRY PACKED)

2 GARLIC CLOVES

⅓ CUP PLAIN NONFAT YOGURT

½ TEASPOON HOT PEPPER SAUCE

SALMON CAKES

1 BAKING POTATO, THINLY SLICED

2 GARLIC CLOVES

ONE 14¾-OUNCE CAN PINK SALMON, DRAINED

2 TABLESPOONS PLUS ½ CUP PLAIN DRIED BREAD CRUMBS

½ CUP MINCED FRESH DILL

1 TABLESPOON CAPERS, RINSED AND DRAINED

1 TABLESPOON OLIVE OIL

For the sauce:

1. Bring a small saucepan of water to a boil. Add the sun-dried tomatoes and 2 garlic cloves and cook for 3 minutes. Reserve ⅓ cup of the cooking liquid for the sauce, then drain the tomatoes and garlic, discarding the remaining liquid.

2. In a food processor, combine the blanched tomatoes and garlic with the reserved cooking liquid, yogurt, and hot pepper sauce. Process the mixture to a smooth purée. Transfer to a bowl and set aside.

For the salmon cakes:

1. Bring a medium saucepan of water to a boil and add 2 garlic cloves and the potato. Cook until the potato is tender, about 6 to 7 minutes. Drain and place in a large bowl. Mash the potato and garlic together using a potato masher. Add the salmon, 2 tablespoons of the bread crumbs, dill, and capers and stir to mix well. Shape the mixture into 8 patties.

2. Heat the olive oil in large nonstick skillet over medium heat. Place the remaining ½ cup bread crumbs on a plate or in a shallow bowl and dredge the salmon cakes in the bread crumbs, coating them on both sides. Place the salmon cakes in the skillet and cook for about 3 minutes on each side, until golden brown and heated through. Serve with the tomato sauce drizzled on top.

Grilled Shrimp Skewers

SERVES 10

▶   CALORIES: **111**
    SODIUM: **169 MILLIGRAMS**

Prep time: **5 minutes**
Cooking time: **5 minutes**

Low in fat and high in protein, shrimp makes a great appetizer for anyone watching their calories. Grilling them on skewers is quick and mess-free, plus it imparts a hint of smoky flavor to the shrimp.

2 TABLESPOONS OLIVE OIL
1 TABLESPOON CHILI POWDER
1 TABLESPOON HONEY
¼ TEASPOON FRESHLY GROUND PEPPER
30 SHRIMP, PEELED, DEVEINED, AND TAILS LEFT ON

1. Preheat a grill or grill pan to medium-high heat. Soak ten wooden skewers in water.

2. In a medium bowl, combine the olive oil, chili powder, honey, and pepper. Add the shrimp and toss to coat.

3. Thread each skewer with 3 shrimp.

4. Cook on the grill for about 2 minutes per side, until the shrimp are pink and cooked through. Serve immediately.

Southwestern-Style Cocktail Meatballs

SERVES 6

▶ CALORIES: **250**
SODIUM: **137 MILLIGRAMS**

Prep time: **10 minutes**
Cooking time: **15 minutes**

Lean ground turkey is mild in flavor, so the flavors of cilantro, jalapeño, and spices shine in these meatballs. Serve them on a platter with toothpicks and a bowl of the dipping sauce on the side for a party dish your guests are sure to love.

MEATBALLS

COOKING SPRAY

1 JALAPEÑO CHILE, SEEDED

2 GARLIC CLOVES

¼ CUP CHOPPED CILANTRO

3 SCALLIONS

1¼ POUNDS LEAN GROUND TURKEY

¼ CUP DRY BREAD CRUMBS

1 EGG

1 TEASPOON GROUND CUMIN

PINCH OF DRIED OREGANO

FRESHLY GROUND PEPPER

DIPPING SAUCE

1 CUP REDUCED-FAT SOUR CREAM

JUICE AND ZEST OF 2 LIMES

¼ CUP FINELY MINCED CILANTRO

For the meatballs:

1. Preheat the oven to 400°F. Spray a large baking sheet lightly with cooking spray.

continued ▶

2. In a food processor, combine the jalapeño, garlic, cilantro, and scallions, and pulse several times until the mixture is finely minced. Transfer to a large bowl and add the turkey, bread crumbs, egg, cumin, oregano, and pepper. Mix well.

3. Shape the mixture into 1½-inch balls and arrange them in a single layer on the prepared baking sheet. Bake in the preheated oven until lightly browned and cooked through, about 15 minutes.

For the dipping sauce:

1. In a small bowl, combine the sour cream, lime zest and juice, and cilantro, and stir to mix well.

2. Serve the meatballs hot with the dipping sauce on the side.

CHAPTER FIVE

Soups and Salads

Quick Pumpkin-Apple Soup

SERVES 4

▶ CALORIES: **246**
SODIUM: **148 MILLIGRAMS**

Prep time: **5 minutes**
Cooking time: **20 minutes**

With their bright orange color, pumpkins deliver abundant beta-carotene. This immunity-boosting soup is beautiful as well as delicious. The sweetness of apple and the spice of ground ginger give it a bit of a twist.

1 TABLESPOON OLIVE OIL
2 SLICES TURKEY BACON, DICED
1 ONION, DICED
ONE 29-OUNCE CAN PURÉED PUMPKIN
3½ CUPS LOW-SODIUM VEGETABLE BROTH
1 CUP UNSWEETENED APPLESAUCE
2 TEASPOONS GROUND GINGER
½ TEASPOON FRESHLY GROUND PEPPER
½ CUP LOW-FAT SOUR CREAM

1. Heat the olive oil in a large stockpot over medium-high heat. Add the bacon and onion and cook, stirring frequently, until the onion is softened and the bacon is crisp, about 5 minutes. Add the pumpkin, broth, applesauce, ginger, and pepper, and bring to a simmer.

2. Cook, uncovered, stirring occasionally, for about 15 minutes.

3. Stir in the sour cream and serve hot.

Green Soup with Goat Cheese

SERVES 4

▶ CALORIES: **21**
SODIUM: **274 MILLIGRAMS**

Prep time: **5 minutes**
Cooking time: **25 minutes**

Calorie for calorie, dark leafy greens represent one of the most concentrated sources of nutrients—such as beta-carotene, vitamins B, C, E, and K, and minerals like iron and magnesium. The soup's rich green hue sends the message of goodness, in the form of spinach, watercress, and sorrel. Naturally low-fat goat cheese adds rich creaminess, while the watercress and sorrel provide pepper and lemon accents. If you can't find sorrel, use more spinach and stir in a couple tablespoons of lemon juice just before serving.

1 TABLESPOON OLIVE OIL

2 LEEKS, GREEN AND LIGHT GREEN PARTS ONLY, THINLY SLICED

2 TABLESPOONS SHERRY

4 CUPS LOW-SODIUM VEGETABLE BROTH

2 CUPS WATER

1 POTATO, PEELED AND DICED

1 POUND SPINACH LEAVES, TOUGH STEMS TRIMMED AND DISCARDED

2 CUPS WATERCRESS

2 CUPS SORREL

¼ TEASPOON CAYENNE

½ CUP CRUMBLED GOAT CHEESE, PLUS MORE FOR GARNISH

2 TABLESPOONS UNSALTED BUTTER

FRESHLY GROUND PEPPER

1. Heat the olive oil in a large stockpot over medium-high heat. Add the leeks and cook, stirring frequently, until the leeks soften, about 5 minutes. Add the sherry and cook, stirring, until the liquid has evaporated.

2. Add the broth, water, and potato and bring to a boil. Reduce the heat to low and simmer, uncovered, for about 15 minutes, until the potato is tender.

continued ▶

3. Stir in spinach, watercress, sorrel, and cayenne. Cook, covered, for about 5 minutes, until the spinach is tender.

4. Remove the pot from the heat, add the goat cheese and butter, and stir until they are well incorporated. Using an immersion blender, or a countertop blender in batches, purée the soup until smooth. Reheat if needed and serve immediately, garnished with a bit of crumbled goat cheese and a generous sprinkling of freshly ground pepper. The soup will keep in the refrigerator for up to 3 days.

Cherry Tomato and Corn Chowder

SERVES 4

▶ CALORIES: **233**
SODIUM: **313 MILLIGRAMS**

Prep time: **10 minutes**
Cooking time: **15 minutes**

Traditional chowders are loaded with calories, fat, and sodium. This quick version uses DASH-friendly substitutions—turkey bacon, low-fat milk, and low-sodium broth—to keep it healthful. Puréeing most of the corn kernels along with low-fat milk makes this chowder thick and satisfying, while the tomatoes give it unmistakable summer flavor and a pretty pop of color. For a vegetarian version, leave out the bacon.

1 TABLESPOON OLIVE OIL
1 ONION, DICED
2 STALKS CELERY, DICED
2 GARLIC CLOVES, MINCED
1 PINT CHERRY TOMATOES, HALVED
2½ CUPS FROZEN CORN KERNELS, THAWED
2 CUPS LOW-FAT MILK
1 TEASPOON CHOPPED FRESH THYME
¼ TEASPOON FRESHLY GROUND PEPPER
1 CUP LOW-SODIUM VEGETABLE OR CHICKEN BROTH
3 SCALLIONS, THINLY SLICED, FOR GARNISH
2 SLICES TURKEY BACON, COOKED AND CRUMBLED, FOR GARNISH (OPTIONAL)

1. Heat the olive oil in a large stockpot over medium-high heat. Add the onion, celery, and garlic and cook, stirring, until the onion is soft, about 5 minutes. Add the tomatoes and cook for 2 or 3 minutes, until the tomatoes just begin to break down.

2. Place 1½ cups of the corn, 1 cup of the milk, the thyme, and pepper in a blender or food processor and process until smooth.

3. Transfer the puréed mixture to the stockpot and bring to a simmer. Add the remaining 1 cup corn and 1 cup milk to the pot along with the broth. Stir well and cook over medium heat for about 5 minutes, until heated through.

4. Serve hot, garnished with the scallions and bacon.

Curried Sweet Potato Soup

SERVES 4

▶ CALORIES: **269**
  SODIUM: **344 MILLIGRAMS**

Prep time: **5 minutes**
Cooking time: **25 minutes**

Sweet potatoes are lauded by nutritionists as one of the most nutrient-dense vegetables. They are loaded with vitamins (B6, C, and D), as well as blood-pressure-lowering minerals like magnesium and potassium. You can tell by their bright orange color that they are also full of beta-carotene, which reduces the risk of many diseases, including cancer, and fights the effects of aging. Here we've spiced them up with curry powder and fresh ginger for a satisfying soup that's perfect for lunch or dinner.

1 TABLESPOON OLIVE OIL
1 ONION, CHOPPED
1½ CUPS LOW-SODIUM VEGETABLE OR CHICKEN BROTH
3 CUPS WATER
2 SWEET POTATOES, PEELED AND DICED
2 CARROTS, PEELED AND SLICED
1 TABLESPOON MINCED FRESH GINGER
1 TABLESPOON CURRY POWDER
FRESHLY GROUND PEPPER

1. Heat the olive oil in large stockpot over medium-high heat. Add the onion and cook, stirring frequently, until soft, about 5 minutes. Add the broth, water, sweet potatoes, carrots, ginger, and curry powder. Bring to a boil and reduce the heat to medium-low. Simmer, uncovered, until the vegetables are tender, about 20 minutes.

2. Using an immersion blender, or in batches in a countertop blender, purée the mixture. If the soup is too thick, add a bit more broth.

3. Reheat the soup, if needed, season with pepper, and serve. The soup will keep covered in the refrigerator for up to a week, and in the freezer for up to three months.

Chinese Egg Drop Soup with Shrimp

SERVES 4

▶ CALORIES: **202**
SODIUM: **424 MILLIGRAMS**

Prep time: **5 minutes**
Cooking time: **15 minutes**

Broth soups are great for filling you up without loading you with fat and calories. This take on classic Chinese egg drop soup gets lots of protein from shrimp and egg. It's full of vitamin-rich veggies like mushrooms, carrots, and peas.

1 TABLESPOON CANOLA OIL
1 CUP SLICED MUSHROOMS
3½ CUPS LOW-SODIUM CHICKEN BROTH
¼ CUP UNSEASONED RICE VINEGAR
2 TABLESPOONS LOW-SODIUM SOY SAUCE
1 TEASPOON GRANULATED SUGAR
1 TEASPOON GRATED FRESH GINGER
12 OUNCES SHRIMP, PEELED AND DEVEINED
¼ CUP FROZEN PEAS
¼ CUP SHREDDED CARROTS
1 TABLESPOON CORNSTARCH MIXED WITH 1 TABLESPOON COLD WATER
1 EGG, LIGHTLY BEATEN

1. Heat the canola oil in a large stockpot over medium-high heat. Add the mushrooms and cook, stirring frequently, until they soften, about 5 minutes.

2. Stir in the broth, vinegar, soy sauce, sugar, and ginger. Bring to a simmer and cook for 2 to 3 minutes. Add the shrimp, peas, and carrots.

3. Bring the soup to a boil and stir in the cornstarch mixture. Keep stirring until the soup thickens and the shrimp are cooked through, about 3 minutes.

4. Stir in the egg and cook, stirring, for 1 or 2 minutes, until the egg is cooked. Serve hot.

Tom Ka Gai (Thai Chicken–Coconut Milk Soup)

SERVES 6

▶ CALORIES: **441**
SODIUM: **419 MILLIGRAMS**

Prep time: **10 minutes**
Cooking time: **20 minutes**

This quick soup is very flavorful and offers a good dose of healthy fats from the coconut oil and coconut milk. Studded with mushrooms, broccoli, and chicken, it is satisfying enough to serve as a meal.

1 TABLESPOON COCONUT OIL

3 SHALLOTS, CHOPPED

2 TEASPOONS THAI RED CURRY PASTE

TWO 14-OUNCE CANS COCONUT MILK

4 CUPS LOW-SODIUM CHICKEN BROTH

1 TABLESPOON HONEY

8 SPRIGS CILANTRO, CHOPPED

8 OUNCES BUTTON OR CREMINI MUSHROOMS, HALVED OR QUARTERED IF LARGE

1 HEAD BROCCOLI, BROKEN INTO FLORETS

2 SKINLESS, BONELESS CHICKEN BREASTS, HALVED LENGTHWISE AND SLICED AGAINST
    THE GRAIN INTO ⅛-INCH-THICK STRIPS

3 TABLESPOONS LIME JUICE

1 TABLESPOON FISH SAUCE

½ CUP MINCED CILANTRO, FOR GARNISH

2 SERRANO CHILES, THINLY SLICED, FOR GARNISH

1 LIME, CUT INTO WEDGES, FOR GARNISH

1. Heat the coconut oil in a large stockpot over medium heat. Add the shallots and cook, stirring frequently, until softened, about 5 minutes. Stir in the curry paste and cook, stirring, for 1 minute. Add the coconut milk, broth, honey, and cilantro, and bring to a boil. Reduce the heat to low and simmer for about 5 minutes.

2. Strain the broth through a fine-mesh sieve, discard the solids, and return the broth to the stockpot over medium heat. Add the mushrooms and broccoli and cook until softened, about 3 minutes. Add the chicken and cook until fully opaque, about 3 minutes.

3. Add the lime juice and fish sauce just before serving. Serve hot, garnished with cilantro, chiles, and lime wedges.

Spicy Chicken-Chipotle Tortilla Soup

SERVES 4

▶ CALORIES: **241**
SODIUM: **173 MILLIGRAMS**

Prep time: **5 minutes**
Cooking time: **15 minutes**

This is classic comfort food with a kick—a healthy chicken soup thickened with crushed tortilla chips and spiced with ground chipotle and cumin. A sprinkling of fresh cilantro is the perfect finishing touch.

1 TABLESPOON OLIVE OIL

1 YELLOW ONION, DICED

2 GARLIC CLOVES, MINCED

12 OUNCES CHICKEN BREAST, DICED

1 TEASPOON GROUND CHIPOTLE

1 TEASPOON GROUND CUMIN

1 CUP WATER

3 CUPS LOW-SODIUM CHICKEN BROTH

ONE 14½-OUNCE CAN NO-SALT-ADDED CRUSHED TOMATOES WITH JUICE

JUICE OF 1 LIME

1 CUP CRUSHED LOW-SODIUM BAKED TORTILLA CHIPS

¼ CUP CHOPPED CILANTRO, FOR GARNISH

1. In a large stockpot, heat the olive oil over medium-high heat. Add the onion and garlic and cook, stirring, until the onion is soft, about 5 minutes. Add the chicken and cook, stirring, for about 2 minutes, until the chicken is opaque. Add the chipotle and cumin and cook for about 30 seconds. Add the water, broth, and tomatoes with juice, and bring to a boil. Reduce the heat to medium, cover, and cook for about 5 minutes. Stir in the lime juice.

2. To serve, divide the crushed tortilla chips among four soup bowls. Ladle the soup over the chips and serve garnished with cilantro.

White Bean and Greens Soup with Sausage

SERVES 6

▶ CALORIES: **232**
SODIUM: **555 MILLIGRAMS**

Prep time: **5 minutes**
Cooking time: **25 minutes**

White beans are an excellent source of protein and are full of fiber and antioxidants. A hefty serving of super-healthy kale adds even more essential vitamins, minerals, fiber, and antioxidants. While cured meats are usually a no-no for those on low-sodium diets, this soup gets a big dose of meaty flavor from a small amount of smoked sausage. With a loaf of crusty bread and a green salad, this hearty soup makes a perfect meal for a cold evening.

2 TABLESPOONS OLIVE OIL
1 ONION, DICED
2 GARLIC CLOVES, MINCED
2 STALKS CELERY, SLICED
2 CARROTS, SLICED
4 OUNCES SPANISH-STYLE CHORIZO OR ANDOUILLE SAUSAGE, DICED
1 BUNCH KALE, CHOPPED
3 CUPS LOW-SODIUM CHICKEN BROTH
1 CUP WATER
ONE 14½-OUNCE CAN NO-SALT-ADDED DICED TOMATOES WITH JUICE
ONE 15-OUNCE CAN WHITE BEANS, SUCH AS CANNELLINI OR GREAT NORTHERN, DRAINED AND RINSED
½ TEASPOON FRESHLY GROUND PEPPER

1. Heat the olive oil in a large stockpot over medium-high heat. Add the onion and garlic and cook, stirring frequently, until the onions are soft, about 5 minutes.

2. Add the celery, carrots, and sausage and cook, stirring occasionally, for 3 minutes. Stir in the kale.

3. Add the broth, water, tomatoes with their juice, beans, and pepper and bring to a boil. Reduce the heat to medium-low and simmer, covered, for about 15 minutes, until the vegetables are soft. Serve hot.

Mixed Baby Greens Salad with Ginger Dressing

SERVES 4

▶ CALORIES: **173**
SODIUM: **200 MILLIGRAMS**

Prep time: **10 minutes**
Cooking time: **None**

This simple, quick salad is full of leafy greens and other healthy veggies like radishes, and the dressing has a kick of ginger. It is perfect on its own as a light meal or served with a spicy Asian stir-fry.

DRESSING

3 TABLESPOONS MINCED ONION

2 TABLESPOONS UNSEASONED RICE VINEGAR

1½ TABLESPOONS FINELY GRATED FRESH GINGER

2 TABLESPOONS CANOLA OIL

1 TABLESPOON KETCHUP

1 TABLESPOON LOW-SODIUM SOY SAUCE

1 TEASPOON SESAME OIL

SALAD

12 OUNCES MIXED BABY GREENS

½ AVOCADO, DICED

½ CUCUMBER, HALVED LENGTHWISE AND THINLY SLICED

4 RADISHES, THINLY SLICED

For the dressing:

In a small bowl, whisk together all the ingredients until well combined.

For the salad:

In a large salad bowl, toss together the ingredients. Add the dressing and toss to coat evenly. Serve immediately.

Asparagus and Edamame Salad with Citrus Vinaigrette

SERVES 4

▶ CALORIES: **339**
SODIUM: **112 MILLIGRAMS**

Prep time: **10 minutes**
Cooking time: **None**

Asparagus is a great source of fiber, antioxidants, vitamins, and minerals. Bright green edamame also comes loaded with fiber, vitamins, and minerals, as well as a good dose of protein. These two bright spring-green vegetables are a foil for the bright pink radishes, sprinkled with Parmesan cheese.

DRESSING

ZEST AND JUICE OF 1 LEMON

1 TABLESPOON WHITE WINE VINEGAR

1 TEASPOON DIJON MUSTARD

1 TEASPOON HONEY

¼ TEASPOON FRESHLY GROUND PEPPER

3 TABLESPOONS OLIVE OIL

SALAD

1 POUND ASPARAGUS, WOODY ENDS SNAPPED OFF AND DISCARDED

2 CUPS SHELLED FROZEN EDAMAME, THAWED

½ BUNCH RADISHES (ABOUT 4 OUNCES), HALVED AND THINLY SLICED

6 HANDFULS BABY ARUGULA

¼ CUP (ABOUT 1 OUNCE) GRATED PARMESAN CHEESE, FOR GARNISH

For the dressing:

In a small bowl, whisk together the lemon zest and juice, vinegar, mustard, honey, and pepper. Whisk in the olive oil until the dressing is well combined and emulsified.

continued ▶

For the salad:

1. Slice the asparagus very thinly (about 1/16 inch) on the diagonal. In a medium bowl, combine the asparagus, edamame, and radishes. Drizzle about three-quarters of the dressing over and toss well to coat.

2. In a medium bowl, combine the arugula with the remaining dressing and toss to coat. Arrange the arugula on four salad plates, top with the asparagus mixture, and serve immediately, garnished with the cheese.

Baby Spinach Salad with Apples, Pecans, and Maple Vinaigrette

SERVES 4

▶ CALORIES: **171**
SODIUM: **115 MILLIGRAMS**

Prep time: **10 minutes**
Cooking time: **None**

One of the most nutrient-dense greens, spinach delivers a good dose of iron, vitamin C, and other nutrients. Paired with pecans and maple vinaigrette, it makes a wonderful fall salad.

¼ CUP MAPLE SYRUP

1 SHALLOT, DICED

2 TABLESPOONS RED WINE VINEGAR

1 TABLESPOON CANOLA OIL

1 TABLESPOON DIJON MUSTARD

1 GARLIC CLOVE, MINCED

¼ TEASPOON FRESHLY GROUND PEPPER

1 CUP SLICED MUSHROOMS

12 OUNCES BABY SPINACH

½ CUP THINLY SLICED RED ONION

½ CUP DICED RED-SKINNED APPLE, SUCH AS BRAEBURN OR GALA

¼ CUP CHOPPED PECANS

1. In a large bowl, whisk together the maple syrup, shallot, vinegar, canola oil, mustard, garlic, and pepper. Add the mushrooms and stir to coat.

2. Add the spinach, onion, apple, and pecans and toss. Serve immediately.

Radicchio, Fennel, and Orange Salad with Olive Vinaigrette

SERVES 4

▶ CALORIES: **152**
  SODIUM: **323 MILLIGRAMS**

Prep time: **10 minutes**
Cooking time: **None**

Fennel contains a unique combination of phytonutrients that give it strong antioxidant properties. Among them is a strong anti-inflammatory compound that has been shown to reduce the risk of cancer. Radicchio is a reddish-purple leafy vegetable with a bitter bite.

VINAIGRETTE

½ TEASPOON ORANGE ZEST

½ CUP ORANGE JUICE

¼ CUP APPLE CIDER VINEGAR

¼ CUP PITTED AND CHOPPED KALAMATA OLIVES

1 TABLESPOON MINCED FRESH OREGANO

1 TEASPOON DIJON MUSTARD

½ TEASPOON FRESHLY GROUND PEPPER

1 TABLESPOON OLIVE OIL

SALAD

3 HEADS RADICCHIO, TORN INTO BITE-SIZE PIECES

2 BULBS FENNEL, TRIMMED AND THINLY SLICED

2 ORANGES (VALENCIA OR NAVEL)

For the dressing:

In a small bowl, whisk together the orange zest, orange juice, vinegar, olives, oregano, mustard, and pepper. Whisk in the olive oil.

For the salad:

1. Toss the radicchio and fennel together in a large salad bowl.

2. Peel the oranges with a sharp knife, making sure to remove all the white pith. Quarter the oranges and thinly slice each quarter crosswise. Add the orange slices to the salad bowl and toss to combine.

3. Drizzle the dressing over the salad and toss well to coat. Serve immediately.

Warm Escarole, Cannellini, and Corn Salad with Pancetta

SERVES 6

▶ CALORIES: **388**
SODIUM: **275 MILLIGRAMS**

Prep time: **5 minutes**
Cooking time: **10 minutes**

Pancetta is Italian bacon. It adds depth of flavor to this hearty salad of fiber-rich white beans, vitamin-rich escarole, and corn.

COOKING SPRAY
2 HEADS ESCAROLE, QUARTERED LENGTHWISE AND RINSED
2 OUNCES PANCETTA, CHOPPED
1 ZUCCHINI, QUARTERED AND CUT INTO JULIENNE STRIPS
1 GARLIC CLOVE, MINCED
1 CUP FRESH CORN KERNELS
ONE 15-OUNCE CAN CANNELLINI BEANS, RINSED AND DRAINED
½ CUP CHOPPED FLAT-LEAF PARSLEY
2 TABLESPOONS RED WINE VINEGAR
1 TEASPOON OLIVE OIL
½ TEASPOON FRESHLY GROUND PEPPER

1. Coat a large nonstick skillet with cooking spray and heat over medium-high heat. Add the escarole and cook, turning on all sides, until wilted, about 3 minutes. Remove the escarole from the pan, trim off the stem end, and roughly chop.

2. Recoat the skillet with cooking spray and heat over medium-high heat. Add the pancetta, zucchini, and garlic and cook until the zucchini softens, about 2 minutes. Stir in the corn and cook for 1 minute.

3. In a large bowl, combine the chopped escarole, pancetta mixture, beans, and parsley. Add the vinegar, olive oil, and pepper, and toss to coat well. Serve immediately.

Lighter Cobb Salad

SERVES 4

▶ CALORIES: **380**
SODIUM: **319 MILLIGRAMS**

Prep time: **15 minutes**
Cooking time: **None**

Traditional Cobb salad is loaded with sodium—not to mention fat and calories—from bacon, blue cheese, and salty dressing. This version uses turkey bacon and includes a small amount of blue cheese in the dressing to distribute the strong flavor. It delivers the same crunchy, salty, tangy flavor and texture, but with much less salt and fat, and fewer calories.

DRESSING

¼ CUP WATER

¼ CUP OLIVE OIL

3 TABLESPOONS WHITE WINE VINEGAR

1 TABLESPOON MINCED SHALLOT

1 TEASPOON DIJON MUSTARD

½ TEASPOON FRESHLY GROUND PEPPER

¼ CUP CRUMBLED BLUE CHEESE

SALAD

1 HEAD ROMAINE LETTUCE, CHOPPED

8 OUNCES COOKED CHICKEN BREAST, DICED OR SHREDDED

2 EGGS, HARD-BOILED, PEELED, AND CHOPPED

2 TOMATOES, DICED

1 CUCUMBER, SEEDED AND SLICED

½ AVOCADO, DICED

2 SLICES COOKED TURKEY BACON, CRUMBLED

continued ▶

Lighter Cobb Salad *continued* ▶

For the dressing:

Whisk together the water, olive oil, vinegar, shallot, mustard, and pepper in a small bowl until well combined. Add the blue cheese and stir to mix.

For the salad:

1. Place the lettuce in a large mixing bowl and drizzle with half of the dressing. Toss to coat. Arrange the lettuce on four serving plates. Top with the rest of the ingredients arranged in rows: chicken, eggs, tomatoes, cucumber, avocado, and bacon.

2. Drizzle the remaining dressing over the salads and serve immediately.

Warm Sweet Potato Salad with Balsamic Vinaigrette

SERVES 6

▶ CALORIES: **257**
SODIUM: **26 MILLIGRAMS**

Prep time: **10 minutes**
Cooking time: **15 minutes**

This salad is a twist on the classic warm potato salad. Replacing white potatoes with sweet potatoes boosts the nutritional content and makes the presentation stunning. Serve this at your next barbecue and you may never go back to the old mayo-and-white-potato version.

2 POUNDS ORANGE-FLESHED SWEET POTATOES, PEELED AND CUT INTO 1-INCH CUBES
3 TABLESPOONS BALSAMIC VINEGAR
1 TABLESPOON CIDER VINEGAR
1 TEASPOON DIJON MUSTARD
½ TEASPOON HONEY
¼ CUP OLIVE OIL
1 STALK CELERY, VERY FINELY DICED
1 TABLESPOON MINCED SHALLOTS
2 TEASPOONS CHOPPED FRESH CHIVES
2 TEASPOONS CHOPPED FLAT-LEAF PARSLEY
½ TEASPOON FRESHLY GROUND PEPPER

1. Place the potatoes in a large pot with water to cover by 3 inches. Bring the water to a boil over high heat. Reduce the heat to medium-low and simmer for about 15 minutes, until the potatoes are tender. Drain and transfer to a large salad bowl.

2. While the potatoes are simmering, make the dressing. In a small bowl, whisk together the balsamic and cider vinegars, mustard, and honey until well combined. Add the olive oil, whisking constantly until the mixture is emulsified. Stir in the celery, shallots, chives, parsley, and pepper.

3. Toss the dressing with the warm potatoes and serve immediately, garnished with more pepper, if desired.

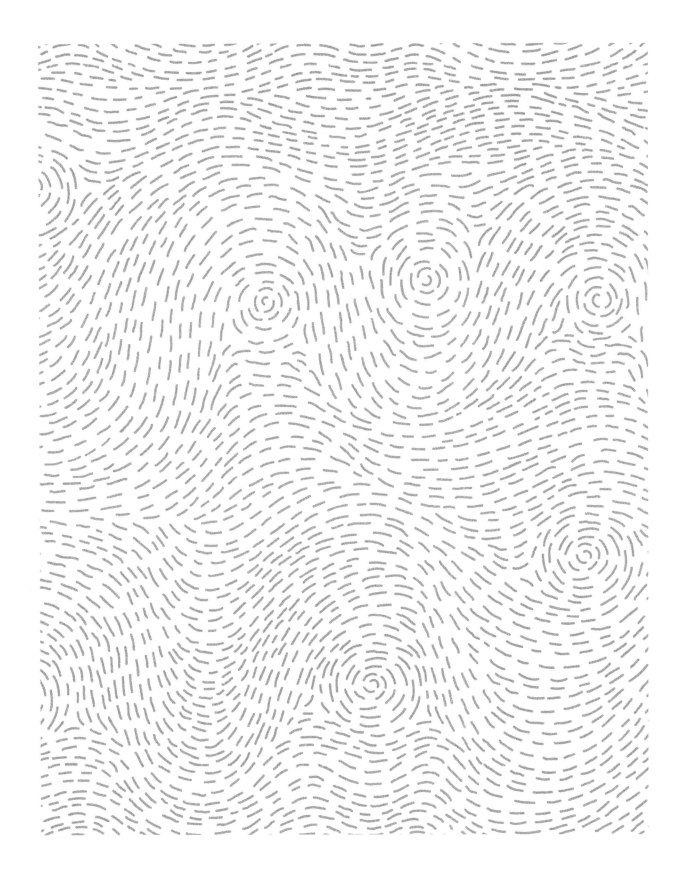

CHAPTER SIX

Entrées

GRILLED MUSHROOM TACOS WITH
  FRESH SALSA

VEGETABLE MU SHU WITH
  WHOLE-WHEAT WRAPS

SPINACH, CHICKPEA, AND SWEET POTATO
  STEW WITH COCONUT MILK

GRILLED HALIBUT WITH TROPICAL
  FRUIT SALSA

SEARED SALMON WITH
  CILANTRO-LIME SAUCE

QUICK SALMON TOSTADAS WITH
  BLACK BEANS AND JALAPEÑOS

PECAN-CRUSTED HONEY-DIJON SALMON

SPICY GRILLED PRAWN SKEWERS WITH
  CUCUMBER-CASHEW SALAD

GREEK TURKEY BURGERS

SPICY STIR-FRIED CHICKEN
  WITH PEANUTS

ARTICHOKE-STUFFED CHICKEN BREASTS
  WITH GOAT CHEESE

WHITE CHICKEN CHILI

PORK CHOPS WITH GREEN
  PEPPERCORN SAUCE

HOISIN PORK AND VEGGIE STIR-FRY

SPICE-RUBBED FLANK STEAK WITH
  TOMATO JAM

SPICY LETTUCE-WRAPPED BEEF

LAMB CHOPS WITH MINTED
  PEA PURÉE

Grilled Mushroom Tacos with Fresh Salsa

SERVES 4

▶ CALORIES: **419**
SODIUM: **224 MILLIGRAMS**

Prep time: **10 minutes**
Cooking time: **15 minutes**

These vegetarian tacos will satisfy big appetites with a wallop of flavor, lots of vitamin C, calcium, and good monounsaturated fat.

3 PLUM TOMATOES, SEEDED AND CHOPPED

½ CUP JULIENNED JICAMA

2 TABLESPOONS CHOPPED CILANTRO

2 TABLESPOONS LIME JUICE

⅛ TEASPOON RED PEPPER FLAKES

1 SERRANO CHILE, MINCED

4 PORTOBELLO MUSHROOM CAPS (ABOUT 1 POUND)

FOUR ¼-INCH-THICK SLICES ONION

1 WHOLE POBLANO CHILE

1 TABLESPOON OLIVE OIL

3 GARLIC CLOVES, THINLY SLICED

½ TEASPOON GROUND CUMIN

8 SIX-INCH CORN TORTILLAS

1 AVOCADO, SLICED

1 CUP (4 OUNCES) SHREDDED REDUCED-FAT CHEDDAR CHEESE

1. Preheat a grill to medium-high heat.

2. In a small bowl, combine the tomatoes, jicama, cilantro, lime juice, red pepper flakes, and serrano chile and mix well.

3. Use a spoon to scrape the gills from the underside of the mushrooms and discard them. Grill the mushrooms, onion, and poblano on the preheated grill until tender, about 5 minutes per side. Seed the poblano, remove the stem, and cut it into thin strips. Cut the mushrooms into thin strips. Chop the onion. Mix the grilled vegetables together in a medium bowl.

4. Heat the olive oil in a large nonstick skillet over medium-high heat. Add the garlic and cook, stirring, for 1 minute. Add the vegetable mixture and the cumin, and cook until thoroughly heated, about 2 minutes.

5. Heat the tortillas according to the package instructions. For each serving, place 2 tortillas on a plate. Top each tortilla with some of the mushroom mixture, the salsa mixture, and a few slices of avocado. Top each taco with about 2 tablespoons of the cheese. Serve immediately.

Vegetable Mu Shu with Whole-Wheat Wraps

SERVES 4

▶   CALORIES: **230**
     SODIUM: **362 MILLIGRAMS**

Prep time: **5 minutes**
Cooking time: **10 minutes**

Using bagged shredded vegetables means this dish can be on the table in no time. Substituting whole-wheat tortillas for the traditional wraps boosts the fiber and nutritional content of this healthy meal.

3 TEASPOONS SESAME OIL

4 EGGS, LIGHTLY BEATEN

2 TEASPOONS MINCED FRESH GINGER

2 GARLIC CLOVES, MINCED

ONE 12-OUNCE BAG SHREDDED COLESLAW VEGGIES OR BROCCOLI SLAW

2 CUPS BEAN SPROUTS

1 BUNCH SCALLIONS, SLICED

1 TABLESPOON LOW-SODIUM SOY SAUCE

1 TABLESPOON UNSEASONED RICE VINEGAR

2 TABLESPOONS HOISIN SAUCE

4 WHOLE-WHEAT TORTILLAS

1. Place a large nonstick skillet over medium heat and add 1 teaspoon of the sesame oil. Add the eggs and cook, stirring, for about 3 minutes, until just set. Transfer the eggs to a plate.

2. In the same skillet, heat the remaining 2 teaspoons sesame oil over medium heat. Add the ginger and garlic and cook for 1 minute. Stir in the shredded vegetables, bean sprouts, half of the scallions, the soy sauce, and vinegar. Cook, covered, for about 3 minutes, until the vegetables are tender. Return the cooked eggs to the pan, add the hoisin sauce and cook, stirring, for about 2 minutes. Remove from the heat and add the remaining scallions.

3. Warm the tortillas according to the package instructions. Place the tortillas on serving plates and divide the vegetable mixture among them. Roll up each tortilla with the veggies tightly inside and serve immediately.

Spinach, Chickpea, and Sweet Potato Stew with Coconut Milk

SERVES 6

▶ CALORIES: **512**
SODIUM: **98 MILLIGRAMS**

Prep time: **5 minutes**
Cooking time: **25 minutes**

This quick and hearty stew is comfort food at its best. It's delicious, creamy, and satisfying, and it's also super healthful, offering vitamins, minerals, antioxidants, healthy fats, and plenty of fiber.

2 TABLESPOONS CANOLA OIL

1 YELLOW ONION, CHOPPED

4 GARLIC CLOVES, MINCED

1 TABLESPOON GRATED FRESH GINGER

ZEST AND JUICE OF 1 LEMON

¼ TEASPOON RED PEPPER FLAKES

2 TABLESPOONS TOMATO PASTE

ONE 15-OUNCE CAN CHICKPEAS, DRAINED AND RINSED

2 SWEET POTATOES, PEELED AND DICED

ONE 14-OUNCE CAN UNSWEETENED COCONUT MILK

1 TEASPOON GROUND GINGER

1 POUND BABY SPINACH

¼ CUP CHOPPED CILANTRO, FOR GARNISH

1. Heat the canola oil in a large stockpot over medium-high heat. Add the onion and cook, stirring occasionally, until the onion is softened and beginning to brown, about 5 minutes.

2. Stir in the garlic, fresh ginger, lemon zest, and red pepper and continue to cook, stirring frequently, for about 3 minutes. Stir in the tomato paste and cook for 1 minute, then add the chickpeas and sweet potatoes.

3. Raise the heat to high and cook for about 3 minutes. Add the coconut milk and ground ginger, stir to mix, and heat until simmering. Reduce the heat to low and cook until the sweet potatoes are tender, about 15 minutes. Add the spinach by the handful, letting it wilt before adding another handful, and cook for a few minutes to ensure that the spinach is fully cooked and warmed through. Stir in the lemon juice.

4. Serve hot, garnished with cilantro.

Grilled Halibut with Tropical Fruit Salsa

SERVES 4

▶ CALORIES: **333**
SODIUM: **202 MILLIGRAMS**

Prep time: **20 minutes** (includes marinating time)
Cooking time: **5 minutes**

Halibut is a meaty and flavorful fish that is loaded with protein as well as blood-pressure-lowering magnesium, vitamins B6 and B12, and omega-3 fatty acids. It's also well suited to grilling, which is one of the quickest healthy cooking methods. This recipe's tropical flavors are perfect for a barbecue on a warm summer evening. A fish-grilling basket is a wise investment. This inexpensive gadget will keep your fish from falling through the slats of the grill and make it easy to flip.

SALSA

1⅓ CUPS DICED PAPAYA OR MANGO (ABOUT 1 POUND)

1 RED BELL PEPPER, DICED

⅓ CUP THINLY SLICED SCALLIONS

¼ CUP LIME JUICE

2 TABLESPOONS CHOPPED CILANTRO

2 JALAPEÑOS, SEEDED AND MINCED

1 GARLIC CLOVE, MINCED

FISH

1 TABLESPOON LEMON JUICE

1 TABLESPOON OLIVE OIL

½ TEASPOON PAPRIKA

1 GARLIC CLOVE, MINCED

½ TEASPOON FRESHLY GROUND PEPPER

FOUR 6-OUNCE SKINLESS HALIBUT FILLETS

COOKING SPRAY

For the salsa:

Add all the ingredients to a medium bowl and stir to combine.

For the fish:

1. In a large, nonreactive baking dish, stir together the lemon juice, olive oil, paprika, garlic, and pepper. Add the fish to the mixture, turn to coat, and let stand for 10 minutes.

2. Spray a grill or grill pan with cooking spray and heat to medium-high heat.

3. Remove the fish from the marinade, discarding the marinade, and place it on the hot grill or grill pan. Cook for about 3 minutes per side, or until the desired degree of doneness is reached. Serve immediately, topped with the salsa.

Seared Salmon with Cilantro-Lime Sauce

SERVES 4

▶ CALORIES: **309**
SODIUM: **79 MILLIGRAMS**

Prep time: **5 minutes**
Cooking time: **15 minutes**

Just one 6-ounce serving of salmon provides more than half the recommended daily allowance of omega-3 fatty acids. Here, it is paired with a bright green sauce that's loaded with flavor. Serve it with sautéed snap peas for a beautiful spring meal.

SAUCE
2 GARLIC CLOVES
1½ CUPS (PACKED) CILANTRO
1 TEASPOON GRATED LIME ZEST
2 TABLESPOONS LIME JUICE
2 TABLESPOONS OLIVE OIL

SALMON
COOKING SPRAY
FOUR 6-OUNCE SALMON FILLETS WITH SKIN
¼ TEASPOON FRESHLY GROUND PEPPER

For the sauce:

Place the garlic in a food processor and pulse to mince. Add the cilantro and lime zest and juice, and pulse until finely chopped. With the food processor running, drizzle in the olive oil until well combined.

For the salmon:

Coat a nonstick skillet with cooking spray and heat it over medium-high heat. Sprinkle the salmon with pepper and place it in the pan skin-side down. Cook until the skin begins to brown, about 5 to 6 minutes. Turn the fish over and cook on the other side until the fish is cooked through and flakes easily with a fork, about 6 minutes. Drizzle with the sauce and serve immediately.

Quick Salmon Tostadas with Black Beans and Jalapeños

SERVES 4

▶ CALORIES: **479**
   SODIUM: **116 MILLIGRAMS**

Prep time: **10 minutes**
Cooking time **15 minutes**

Canned salmon is both convenient and easy on the budget, and offers the same health benefits as fresh does. Made with ingredients you're likely to have in your pantry, these quick tostadas are an easy and delicious weeknight dinner.

EIGHT 6-INCH CORN TORTILLAS

COOKING SPRAY

ONE 6- TO 7-OUNCE CAN BONELESS, SKINLESS WILD ALASKAN SALMON, DRAINED

1 AVOCADO, DICED

2 TABLESPOONS MINCED PICKLED JALAPEÑOS, PLUS 2 TABLESPOONS OF THE PICKLING JUICE

2 CUPS SHREDDED CABBAGE

2 TABLESPOONS CHOPPED CILANTRO

ONE 15-OUNCE CAN BLACK BEANS, RINSED AND DRAINED

3 TABLESPOONS REDUCED-FAT SOUR CREAM

2 TABLESPOONS PREPARED SALSA

2 SCALLIONS, CHOPPED

LIME WEDGES, FOR GARNISH

1. Preheat the oven to 375°F. Position the racks in the upper and lower third of the oven.

2. Spray the tortillas on both sides with cooking spray and arrange them on two baking sheets in a single layer. Bake, rotating and flipping once, until they begin to turn golden, about 12 minutes.

3. Meanwhile, in a medium bowl, stir together the salmon, avocado, and jalapeños.

4. In a another medium bowl, toss together the cabbage, cilantro, and pickling juice.

continued ▶

Quick Salmon Tostadas with Black Beans and Jalapeños *continued* ▶

5. In a food processor, combine the beans, sour cream, salsa, and scallions, and process until smooth. Transfer the purée to a microwave-safe bowl, cover, and cook on high in the microwave for about 2 minutes, until the mixture is hot.

6. To serve, spread some of the bean mixture on each tortilla. Top with some of the salmon mixture. Place a handful of cabbage slaw on top. Serve garnished with lime wedges.

Pecan-Crusted Honey-Dijon Salmon

SERVES 6

▶ CALORIES: **285**
SODIUM: **205 MILLIGRAMS**

Prep time: **5 minutes**
Cooking time: **15 minutes**

This healthy salmon dish, coated with a pecan–bread crumb mixture takes less than 20 minutes to prepare, making it a perfect choice for a busy workday evening. Serve it with quickly sautéed green beans or steamed broccoli and quinoa.

COOKING SPRAY
3 TABLESPOONS DIJON MUSTARD
1 TABLESPOON OLIVE OIL
1 TABLESPOON HONEY
½ CUP FINELY CHOPPED PECANS
½ CUP FRESH BREAD CRUMBS
SIX 4-OUNCE SALMON FILLETS
1 TABLESPOON MINCED FLAT-LEAF PARSLEY, FOR GARNISH

1. Preheat the oven to 400°F. Spray a large baking dish lightly with cooking spray.

2. In a small bowl, combine the mustard, olive oil, and honey. In another small bowl, combine the pecans and bread crumbs.

3. Arrange the fillets in a single layer in the prepared baking dish. Brush each fillet first with the honey-mustard mixture, then top evenly with the pecan mixture.

4. Bake in the preheated oven until the salmon is cooked through and flakes easily with a fork, about 15 minutes. Serve immediately, garnished with parsley.

Spicy Grilled Prawn Skewers with Cucumber-Cashew Salad

SERVES 4

► CALORIES: **420**
SODIUM: **426 MILLIGRAMS**

Prep time: **10 minutes**
Cooking time: **6 minutes**

Low-caloric, quick-cooking prawns are well suited to grilling. Here they get a spicy rub and are served atop a refreshing cucumber salad to cool the fire. This is a perfect meal for a backyard barbecue.

CUCUMBER SALAD

2 CUCUMBERS, PEELED, SEEDED, AND DICED

½ CUP COARSELY CHOPPED UNSALTED ROASTED CASHEWS

2 SCALLIONS, THINLY SLICED

1 TABLESPOON LEMON JUICE

2 TABLESPOONS OLIVE OIL

¼ CUP CHOPPED FLAT-LEAF PARSLEY

GRILLED PRAWN SKEWERS

1 SERRANO CHILE, SEEDED AND FINELY MINCED

1 TABLESPOON OLIVE OIL

1 TEASPOON GROUND CUMIN

1 TEASPOON CHILI POWDER

1½ POUNDS PRAWNS, PEELED AND DEVEINED

Preheat the grill to medium-high. Soak four wooden skewers in water.

For the salad:

In a large bowl, toss together the cucumbers, cashews, scallions, lemon juice, olive oil, and parsley.

For the prawn skewers:

1. In a large bowl, combine the serrano chile, olive oil, cumin, and chili powder. Add the prawns to the bowl and toss to coat with the spice mixture. Thread the prawns onto the skewers.

2. Grill the prawns for about 3 minutes per side, until they are pink and cooked through.

3. To serve, divide the cucumber salad among four serving plates. Top each with a skewer and serve immediately.

Greek Turkey Burgers

SERVES 4

▶ CALORIES: **343**
SODIUM: **309 MILLIGRAMS**

Prep time: **10 minutes**
Cooking time: **10 minutes**

This healthy take on the hamburger gives you all the flavors of a Greek salad and all the fun of a burger in one low-calorie, low-sodium sandwich.

1¼ POUNDS LEAN GROUND TURKEY

1 EGG, BEATEN

½ RED ONION, MINCED

2 TABLESPOONS CHOPPED FLAT-LEAF PARSLEY

2 TABLESPOONS MINCED KALAMATA OLIVES

2 TEASPOONS CHOPPED FRESH OREGANO

1 GARLIC CLOVE, MINCED

½ TEASPOON FRESHLY GROUND PEPPER

4 WHOLE-WHEAT HAMBURGER BUNS, TOASTED

4 HANDFULS BABY SPINACH LEAVES

1 TOMATO, SLICED

4 THIN SLICES RED ONION

1. In a large mixing bowl, combine the turkey, egg, onion, parsley, olives, oregano, garlic, and pepper, and mix well. Shape the mixture into 4 burgers about ½ inch thick.

2. Heat a barbecue, grill, or nonstick skillet over medium-high heat. Cook the burgers for about 4 minutes per side, until cooked through and browned on the outside.

3. Serve the burgers on the toasted buns and garnish with spinach, tomato, and red onion.

Spicy Stir-Fried Chicken with Peanuts

SERVES 4

▶ CALORIES: **263**
SODIUM: **134 MILLIGRAMS**

Prep time: **5 minutes**
Cooking time: **10 minutes**

Stir-fry dishes make great weeknight dinners because they're quick to prepare and usually include protein and veggies in one pan. Just add some steamed brown rice or quinoa, and dinner is served.

SAUCE

3 TABLESPOONS LOW-SODIUM CHICKEN BROTH

1 TABLESPOON TOMATO PASTE

2 TEASPOONS UNSEASONED RICE VINEGAR

1 TEASPOON GRANULATED SUGAR

1 TEASPOON LOW-SODIUM SOY SAUCE

½ TEASPOON SESAME OIL

¼ TEASPOON CORNSTARCH

¼ TEASPOON RED PEPPER FLAKES, PLUS MORE TO TASTE

CHICKEN

1 POUND SKINLESS, BONELESS CHICKEN BREAST, CUT INTO 1-INCH CUBES

1 TEASPOON CHINESE RICE WINE, DRY SHERRY, OR DRY WHITE WINE

1 TEASPOON LOW-SODIUM SOY SAUCE

1½ TEASPOONS CORNSTARCH

½ TEASPOON MINCED GARLIC

1 TABLESPOON CANOLA OIL

TWO ½-INCH-THICK SLICES GINGER, SMASHED

2 CUPS SUGAR SNAP PEAS

¼ CUP UNSALTED DRY-ROASTED PEANUTS, FOR GARNISH

1 SCALLION, THINLY SLICED, FOR GARNISH

continued ▶

For the sauce:

In a small bowl, whisk together the broth, tomato paste, vinegar, sugar, soy sauce, sesame oil, cornstarch, and red pepper flakes.

For the chicken:

1. In a medium bowl, mix together the chicken, wine, soy sauce, cornstarch, and garlic, and stir to coat the chicken thoroughly.

2. Heat a large skillet over high heat and add the canola oil. Add the ginger and cook, stirring, for 10 seconds. Add the chicken, spreading it out into a single layer. Cook without disturbing for about 1 minute, just until the chicken begins to brown. Continue to cook, stirring, for 30 seconds, then spread the chicken out again into a single layer and cook for 30 seconds. Continue cooking the chicken while stirring for 1 or 2 minutes, until the chicken is lightly browned all over. Stir in the snap peas and cook for 1 minute. Add the sauce and cook, stirring, for about 1 minute, until the sauce thickens and becomes glossy.

3. Serve immediately, garnished with the peanuts and scallions.

Artichoke-Stuffed Chicken Breasts with Goat Cheese

SERVES 4

▶ CALORIES: **316**
    SODIUM: **202 MILLIGRAMS**

Prep time: **10 minutes**
Cooking time: **20 minutes**

The humble-looking artichoke is one of the most antioxidant-rich foods around and is full of fiber, folate, and vitamins C and K. Goat cheese and lemon are perfect flavor partners; together they turn plain chicken breast into a feast.

ONE 6-OUNCE JAR MARINATED ARTICHOKE HEARTS, DRAINED AND CHOPPED
ONE 3-OUNCE PACKAGE HERBED GOAT CHEESE, AT ROOM TEMPERATURE
2½ TABLESPOONS WHOLE-WHEAT BREAD CRUMBS
2 TEASPOONS ITALIAN SEASONING
2 TEASPOONS GRATED LEMON ZEST
¼ TEASPOON FRESHLY GROUND PEPPER
FOUR 6-OUNCE SKINLESS, BONELESS CHICKEN BREAST HALVES
COOKING SPRAY

1. Preheat the oven to 375°F.

2. In a medium bowl, stir together the artichoke hearts, goat cheese, bread crumbs, Italian seasoning, lemon zest, and pepper.

3. Place one chicken breast on a piece of plastic wrap on top of a sturdy work surface. Top it with another piece of plastic wrap and, using a meat tenderizing mallet or a rolling pin, pound it to an even thickness of about ¼ inch. Repeat with each remaining chicken breast.

4. Place about 2 tablespoons of the artichoke-cheese mixture on one end of each of the chicken pieces and roll the chicken up around it. Secure with toothpicks.

5. Coat a large, oven-safe skillet with cooking spray and heat it over medium-high heat. Brown the chicken on both sides, cooking it for about 3 minutes per side. Transfer the skillet to the preheated oven and bake until the chicken is cooked through, about 15 minutes. Remove the chicken from the pan and let rest for 5 minutes. Slice each breast in half crosswise and transfer to a serving plate. Serve immediately.

White Chicken Chili

SERVES 4

▶ CALORIES: **485**
SODIUM: **149 MILLIGRAMS**

Prep time: **5 minutes**
Cooking time: **25 minutes**

If you crave the hearty flavor of chili, but are intent on keeping excess fat and calories out of your diet, white chicken chili is the dish for you. Garnish this spicy version with diced avocado, fresh salsa, sour cream, shredded cheese, or tortilla chips as desired. Chili is one of those dishes that gets better with time. Make a double batch and store the extra in a sealed container in the refrigerator for up to 3 days, or in the freezer for up to 3 months.

1 TABLESPOON CANOLA OIL

1 ONION, CHOPPED

3 GARLIC CLOVES, MINCED

1 TO 3 JALAPEÑOS, SEEDED AND DICED

2 TEASPOONS GROUND CUMIN

1½ TEASPOONS GROUND CORIANDER

1 TEASPOON CHILI POWDER

1 TEASPOON DRIED OREGANO

¼ TO ½ TEASPOON CAYENNE

4 CUPS LOW-SODIUM CHICKEN BROTH

3 CUPS CHOPPED COOKED CHICKEN BREAST

THREE 15-OUNCE CANS WHITE BEANS

¼ CUP CHOPPED CILANTRO, FOR GARNISH

1. Heat the canola oil in a large stockpot over medium heat. Add the onion and garlic, and cook, stirring frequently, until the onion is soft, about 5 minutes. Add the jalapeño, cumin, coriander, chili powder, oregano, and cayenne. Cook, stirring frequently, for 2 to 3 minutes, until the jalapeño begins to soften.

2. Add the broth, chicken, and beans, and bring to a boil over medium-high heat. Reduce the heat to medium-low and simmer, uncovered, stirring occasionally, for about 15 minutes. Serve hot, garnished with cilantro.

Pork Chops with Green Peppercorn Sauce

▶ CALORIES: **370**
SODIUM: **290 MILLIGRAMS**

Prep time: **5 minutes**
Cooking time: **10 minutes**

Green peppercorns are simply black peppercorns that have been harvested before they are ripe. They are usually sold in jars with brine, and they have an unusual sharp and tangy flavor. You can find green peppercorns in most supermarkets in the pickle section, but you can substitute a teaspoon of cracked black peppercorns in this dish if you prefer.

FOUR 4-OUNCE BONELESS PORK CHOPS, ½ INCH THICK, TRIMMED

½ TEASPOON FRESHLY GROUND PEPPER

3 TABLESPOONS ALL-PURPOSE FLOUR

2 TABLESPOONS OLIVE OIL

1 SHALLOT, MINCED

1 GARLIC CLOVE, SMASHED

½ CUP BRANDY

¼ CUP REDUCED-FAT SOUR CREAM

2 TABLESPOONS LOW-SODIUM CHICKEN BROTH

2 TABLESPOONS GREEN PEPPERCORNS IN BRINE, DRAINED

1. Dust the pork chops on both sides with pepper and dredge them in the flour.

2. Heat the olive oil in a large skillet over medium-high heat. Add the pork chops (you may have to cook the chops in two batches to avoid crowding the pan), and cook, turning once, until browned and cooked through, about 3 minutes on each side. Place the cooked chops on a plate and cover loosely with aluminum foil.

continued ▶

Pork Chops with Green Peppercorn Sauce *continued* ▶

3. Reduce the heat to medium-low. Add the shallot and garlic to the pan, and cook, stirring frequently, until the shallot is softened, about 3 minutes.

4. Add the brandy to the pan and cook, stirring frequently, for 2 minutes, until most of the brandy has evaporated. Stir in the sour cream, broth, and green peppercorns. Simmer, stirring, until the sauce is thickened and well combined.

5. Serve the pork chops immediately with the sauce spooned over the top.

Hoisin Pork and Veggie Stir-Fry

SERVES 4

▶ CALORIES: **390**
SODIUM: **383 MILLIGRAMS**

Prep time: **15 minutes**
Cooking time: **15 minutes**

This classic savory-sweet sauce flavors the lean pork tenderloin and veggies for a one-pot meal that is sure to become a favorite. Serve over steamed brown rice for a complete meal.

¼ CUP HOISIN SAUCE

1 TABLESPOON MIRIN (JAPANESE RICE WINE), DRY SHERRY, OR DRY WHITE WINE

1 TABLESPOON SESAME OIL

1 TABLESPOON GRATED FRESH GINGER

2 GARLIC CLOVES, MINCED

1½ POUNDS PORK TENDERLOIN, THINLY SLICED

2 TABLESPOONS SESAME SEEDS

2 TEASPOONS SESAME OIL

1 SHALLOT, THINLY SLICED

1 CUP SNOW PEAS, SLICED ON THE DIAGONAL

2 CUPS SHREDDED CHINESE CABBAGE

1 RED BELL PEPPER, CUT INTO MATCHSTICK PIECES

1 TABLESPOON CORNSTARCH MIXED WITH 1 TABLESPOON COLD WATER

4 SCALLIONS, TRIMMED AND THINLY SLICED ON THE DIAGONAL, FOR GARNISH

1. In a large bowl, stir together the hoisin sauce, wine, sesame oil, ginger, and garlic. Add the pork and toss to coat well. Let sit for 15 minutes.

2. Toast the sesame seeds in a large skillet over medium heat until they become fragrant, about 2 to 3 minutes. Transfer to a bowl and set aside.

3. Remove the pork from the marinade, reserving the marinade.

continued ▶

Hoisin Pork and Veggie Stir-Fry *continued* ▶

4. Add the sesame oil to the skillet and heat over medium-high heat. Add the shallot and cook, stirring, until it begins to soften, about 3 minutes. Add the pork and cook, stirring, for 1 minute. Add the snow peas, cabbage, and bell pepper, and cook, stirring, until the vegetables begin to soften, about 3 minutes. Stir in the reserved marinade and bring to a boil. Cook, stirring, until the sauce begins to thicken, about 3 minutes. Add the cornstarch mixture and cook, stirring, until the sauce has thickened, about 2 minutes. Serve immediately, garnished with the scallions and toasted sesame seeds.

Spice-Rubbed Flank Steak with Tomato Jam

SERVES 8

▶ CALORIES: **266**
SODIUM: **71 MILLIGRAMS**

Prep time: **10 minutes**
Cooking time: **20 minutes**

Lean flank steak satisfies a red-meat craving and provides a good dose of iron. The spice rub gives the dish a kick, and tomato jam adds a sweet finish. The jam can be made ahead and stored in the refrigerator for up to a week. Bring it to room temperature before serving.

TOMATO JAM

6 TOMATOES (ABOUT 4 POUNDS), CORED AND CUT IN HALF CROSSWISE

⅓ CUP GRANULATED SUGAR

⅓ CUP GRATED ONION

3 GARLIC CLOVES, MINCED

2 JALAPEÑOS, SEEDED AND MINCED

¼ CUP CHOPPED CILANTRO

3 TABLESPOONS LIME JUICE

STEAK

1 TEASPOON GROUND CUMIN

2 TEASPOONS GROUND CORIANDER

1 TEASPOON PAPRIKA

1 TEASPOON FRESHLY GROUND PEPPER

1 TEASPOON SALT-FREE GARLIC POWDER

½ TEASPOON CAYENNE

2 POUNDS FLANK STEAK, TRIMMED

continued ▶

Heat a grill or grill pan to high heat.

For the tomato jam:

Mince the tomatoes and place them with their juice in a medium saucepan. Add the sugar, onion, garlic, and jalapeños, and bring to a boil over medium-high heat. Reduce the heat to medium-low and simmer, stirring occasionally, for about 20 minutes, until the mixture is reduced to about 2 cups. Remove from the heat and let cool.

For the steak:

1. While the jam is simmering, in a small bowl, combine the cumin, coriander, paprika, pepper, garlic powder, and cayenne. Rub the spice mixture all over the steak on both sides.

2. Place the steak on the grill and cook for about 3 minutes per side for medium-rare (4 or 5 minutes for more well done). Remove from the heat and let rest for 5 minutes before slicing.

3. Stir the cilantro and lime juice into the jam right before serving with the steak.

4. To serve, slice the steak diagonally across the grain into ¼-inch-thick slices. Serve the sliced steak immediately, garnished with a dollop of the jam.

Spicy Lettuce-Wrapped Beef

SERVES 4

▶ CALORIES: **287**
SODIUM: **336 MILLIGRAMS**

Prep time: **15 minutes**
Cooking time: **15 minutes**

This is a fun, do-it-yourself dish for a family dinner or casual dinner party. Serve with bowls of extra condiments, like chopped fresh herbs, sliced chiles, chili paste, Asian-style pickles, or kimchi, if you like.

1 POUND FLANK STEAK

¼ TEASPOON FRESHLY GROUND PEPPER

½ CUCUMBER, PEELED AND DICED

6 CHERRY TOMATOES, HALVED

1 SHALLOT, THINLY SLICED

1 TABLESPOON FINELY CHOPPED FRESH MINT

1 TABLESPOON FINELY CHOPPED FRESH BASIL

1 TABLESPOON FINELY CHOPPED CILANTRO

1 TABLESPOON BROWN SUGAR

2 TABLESPOONS LOW-SODIUM SOY SAUCE

2 TABLESPOONS LIME JUICE

½ TEASPOON RED PEPPER FLAKES

1 HEAD BIBB LETTUCE, LEAVES SEPARATED

1. Preheat a grill or grill pan to medium-high heat.

2. Sprinkle the steak with pepper on both sides.

3. Grill the steak, turning once, until the desired degree of doneness has been reached, about 7 minutes per side for medium rare. Transfer the steak to a cutting board, cover loosely with foil, and let rest for 5 minutes. Cut into ¼-inch-thick slices, cutting across the grain.

continued ▶

4. In a large bowl, mix together the sliced steak, cucumber, tomatoes, shallot, mint, basil, and cilantro. In a small bowl, whisk together the sugar, soy sauce, lime juice, and red pepper flakes, and pour the mixture over the steak mixture and toss to coat.

5. To serve, place the meat mixture in a serving bowl with a large spoon. Set the lettuce leaves on a serving plate and instruct diners to scoop some of the meat into a lettuce leaf, wrap it up like a burrito, and enjoy.

Lamb Chops with Minted Pea Purée

SERVES 4

▶ CALORIES: **463**
SODIUM: **205 MILLIGRAMS**

Prep time: **10 minutes**
Cooking time: **20 minutes**

Both peas and lamb symbolize the arrival of spring. Lamb is loaded with iron and zinc, while peas contain both omega-3 and omega-6 fatty acids, which help our bodies absorb important nutrients.

4 TEASPOONS OLIVE OIL

3 GARLIC CLOVES, MINCED

2 CUPS FROZEN PEAS (ABOUT 12 OUNCES), THAWED

¾ CUP WATER, PLUS MORE AS NEEDED

½ TEASPOON FRESHLY GROUND PEPPER

8 LAMB LOIN CHOPS (ABOUT 1½ POUNDS), TRIMMED

1 TABLESPOON CHOPPED FRESH MINT

1. Preheat the oven to 375°F.

2. Heat 2 teaspoons of the olive oil in a medium saucepan set over medium heat. Add the garlic and cook, stirring constantly, for 1 minute. Add the peas and water and bring to a boil. Lower the heat, cover, and simmer for 5 minutes. Remove the pan from the heat.

3. Sprinkle both sides of the lamb chops with the pepper. Heat the remaining 2 teaspoons of olive oil over medium-high heat in a large, oven-safe skillet. Add the lamb chops and cook for about 2 minutes on one side, until browned on the bottom. Turn the chops over and transfer the skillet to the preheated oven.

4. Bake 8 to 12 minutes for medium rare, or a bit longer for more well done.

5. While the meat is in the oven, put the pea mixture in a food processor. Add the mint and pulse to a coarse purée. If the mixture is too thick, add a bit more water, 1 tablespoon at a time, to thin it.

6. Spoon some of the purée onto each of four serving plates and top each with 2 lamb chops. Serve immediately.

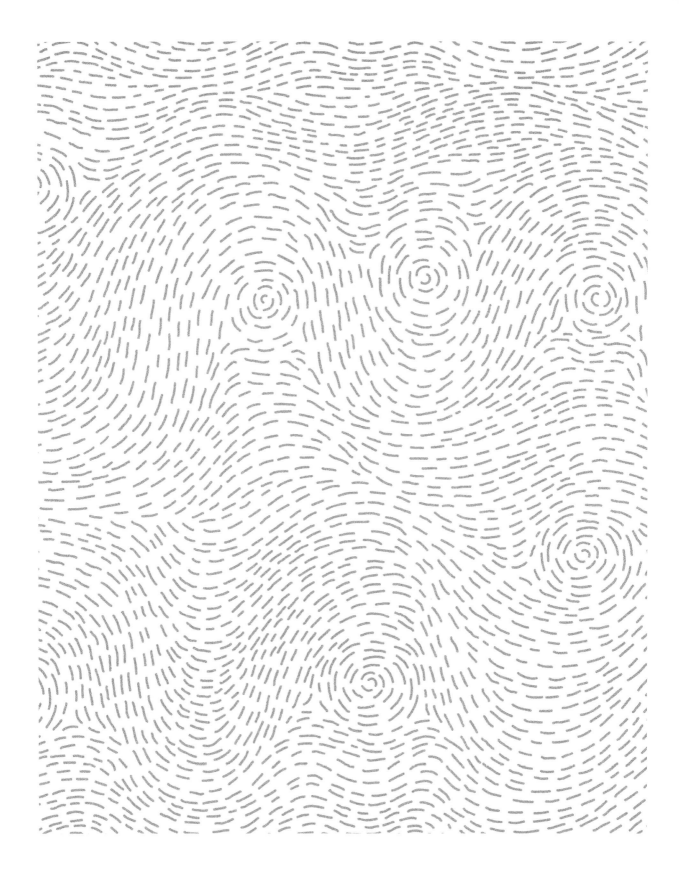

CHAPTER SEVEN

Desserts

Fruit Salad with Fresh Mint

SERVES 4

▶ CALORIES: **122**
SODIUM: **23 MILLIGRAMS**

Prep time: **30 minutes** (includes standing time)
Cooking time: **None**

This refreshing salad provides a great deal of energy for your busy day, with gorgeous colors and different textures. Use ripe but firm fruit for the best results, and be sure to let the salad stand for at least 20 minutes so the mint has time to blend with the other ingredients.

½ CANTALOUPE, PEELED, SEEDED, AND CUT INTO ½-INCH PIECES
¼ HONEYDEW MELON, PEELED, SEEDED, AND CUT INTO ½-INCH PIECES
1 CUP FRESH BLUEBERRIES
1 CUP SLICED FRESH STRAWBERRIES
1 ASIAN PEAR, CUT INTO ½-INCH PIECES
½ CUP ORANGE JUICE
4 TABLESPOONS CHOPPED FRESH MINT

1. In a large serving bowl, toss together the cantaloupe, honeydew, blueberries, strawberries, and pear.

2. In a small bowl, combine the orange juice and mint. Pour the juice over the fruit and toss to coat.

3. Let stand for about 20 minutes, tossing a few times to blend the flavors. Serve at room temperature.

Mixed Berry Meringue Soufflé

SERVES 6

▶   CALORIES: **170**
    SODIUM: **28 MILLIGRAMS**

Prep time: **15 minutes**
Cooking time: **10 minutes**

These airy soufflés, streaked with deep red berries, are a wonder to see. Who would believe they are so easy to make, low-fat, low-calorie, and incredibly delicious?

4 CUPS DICED BERRIES (STRAWBERRIES, RASPBERRIES, BLUEBERRIES, BLACKBERRIES,
   OR A COMBINATION)
¼ CUP WATER
⅓ CUP PLUS ½ CUP GRANULATED SUGAR
1 TABLESPOON CORNSTARCH MIXED WITH 1 TABLESPOON COLD WATER
1 TEASPOON VANILLA EXTRACT
3 EGG WHITES
¼ TEASPOON CREAM OF TARTAR

1. Preheat the oven to 400°F.

2. In a medium saucepan over medium heat, combine the berries with ¼ cup water and ⅓ cup of the sugar and bring to a simmer, stirring frequently. Add the cornstarch mixture to the simmering berries and cook, stirring, until thickened, about 1 minute. Mix in the vanilla and remove from the heat.

3. In a large bowl, beat the egg whites with an electric mixer fitted with a whisk attachment and set on medium-high speed until soft peaks form, about 3 minutes. Gradually add the remaining ½ cup sugar and cream of tartar and continue beating until stiff, glossy peaks form. Spoon about ½ cup of the berry mixture into the egg mixture and swirl it in using a rubber spatula.

4. Spoon the rest of the berry mixture into six 6-ounce ramekins set on a baking sheet. Mound the egg mixture on top of the fruit, using your fingertips to swirl it into pretty peaks. Bake in the preheated oven until the peaks begin to turn golden, about 5 minutes. Serve warm.

Port-Roasted Red Cherries with Vanilla Whipped "Cream"

SERVES 4

▶   CALORIES: **220**
SODIUM: **52 MILLIGRAMS**

Prep time: **10 minutes**
Cooking time: **15 minutes**

Deep red cherries pair beautifully with a ruby port. Topped with a vanilla-scented whipped topping (you'd never guess it's low-fat), this dessert makes a sophisticated finish to an elegant meal.

FRUIT
COOKING SPRAY
1 POUND RED CHERRIES, PITTED AND HALVED
2 TABLESPOONS GRANULATED SUGAR
¼ CUP RUBY PORT

WHIPPED TOPPING
1 EGG WHITE
2 TABLESPOONS GRANULATED SUGAR
¼ TEASPOON CREAM OF TARTAR
¼ CUP LOW-FAT EVAPORATED MILK, CHILLED
½ TEASPOON VANILLA EXTRACT

Preheat the oven to 450°F. Spray four 8-ounce ramekins with cooking spray and place them on a baking sheet.

For the fruit:

Place the cherries evenly in the prepared ramekins, and sprinkle them with the sugar. Cook in the preheated oven until the cherries soften and become juicy, about 10 minutes. Remove the ramekins from the oven and drizzle 1 tablespoon port into each. Stir to coat the cherries. Return the pan to the oven and cook until the liquid begins to bubble and thicken, about 5 minutes.

For the topping:

1. While the cherries are roasting, place the egg white and sugar in the top of a double boiler over simmering water and heat gently, whisking constantly, until the mixture is warm and the sugar is completely dissolved. Test this by dipping your fingers into the mixture. If the mixture feels smooth, not grainy, it is done.

2. Transfer to a mixing bowl. Add the cream of tartar and beat with an electric mixer fitted with a whisk attachment until stiff peaks form, about 3 minutes. Whisk in the evaporated milk and vanilla. Beat until the mixture holds soft peaks, about 3 minutes.

3. Serve the cherries warm, topped with a dollop of the whipped topping.

Broiled Figs with Coconut-Honey Caramel

SERVES 4 TO 6

▶ CALORIES: **303**
SODIUM: **16 MILLIGRAMS**

Prep time: **5 minutes**
Cooking time: **15 minutes**

This simple dessert features healthy ingredients, but tastes sinfully decadent all the same. Try it with apples, pears, or peaches, depending on what's in season.

CARAMEL
1 CUP COCONUT MILK
½ CUP HONEY
2 TABLESPOONS PALM SUGAR

FIGS
12 FRESH FIGS, TRIMMED AND HALVED
1 TABLESPOON COCONUT OIL
¼ TEASPOON GROUND CINNAMON

Preheat the broiler to high.

For the caramel:

Combine the coconut milk, honey, and palm sugar in a medium saucepan over medium-high heat. Bring almost to a boil, stirring frequently. Cook, stirring, for about 10 minutes, until the sauce becomes very thick and dark.

For the figs:

1. Place them cut-side up on a baking sheet and brush with the coconut oil. Place under the broiler and cook until they begin to caramelize, about 3 to 4 minutes.

2. Remove the figs from the broiler and place on serving plates. Drizzle with the caramel and sprinkle with the cinnamon. Serve immediately.

Apple Phyllo Triangles

SERVES 6

▶ CALORIES: **94**
SODIUM: **93 MILLIGRAMS**

Prep time: **15 minutes**
Cooking time: **15 minutes**

Crisp phyllo dough magically transforms a handful of simple ingredients—apples, raisins, and brown sugar—into a seemingly decadent dessert. Most phyllo desserts are drenched in butter, but this is lightened up significantly by using cooking spray instead.

COOKING SPRAY
1 APPLE, PEELED AND DICED SMALL
2 TABLESPOONS RAISINS
2 TABLESPOONS LIGHT BROWN SUGAR
SIX 9-BY-14-INCH SHEETS PHYLLO DOUGH (THAWED)

1. Preheat the oven to 375°F. Spray a baking sheet with cooking spray.

2. Mix the apple, raisins, and brown sugar together in a medium bowl.

3. To assemble the triangles, lay a sheet of phyllo dough on a work surface and spritz it all over with cooking spray. Place a second sheet of phyllo dough on top and spray it with cooking spray. Repeat with a third sheet of phyllo dough. Cut the stack lengthwise into 3 long strips, using kitchen shears or a sharp knife.

4. On the first strip, place a rounded tablespoon of the filling at one end, leaving about 2 inches uncovered at the end. Fold the end over the filling at a 45-degree angle (like folding a flag). Continue folding end over end to form an enclosed triangular bundle. Repeat with the other two strips and set the triangles on a baking sheet. Repeat the process to make 3 more triangles with the remaining 3 sheets of phyllo and the rest of the filling.

5. Spritz the triangles with cooking spray and bake in the preheated oven until lightly browned and crisp, about 15 minutes. Serve warm or at room temperature.

Banana-Nut Wontons with Bourbon Caramel

SERVES 8

▶ CALORIES: **160**
SODIUM: **110 MILLIGRAMS**

Prep time: **10 minutes**
Cooking time: **15 minutes**

Wonton wrappers are a low-fat, low-calorie substitute for butter-laden puff pastry. The delicate wrappers make the banana, pecans, and caramel the stars of the show. Bananas add blood-pressure-lowering magnesium and potassium.

WONTONS

COOKING SPRAY

1 BANANA, DICED

¼ CUP PECAN PIECES

2 TABLESPOONS BROWN SUGAR

1 EGG, BEATEN

16 SQUARE OR ROUND WONTON WRAPPERS

CARAMEL

1 TABLESPOON UNSALTED BUTTER

⅓ CUP BROWN SUGAR

2 TABLESPOONS BOURBON OR OTHER WHISKEY

6 TABLESPOONS WHOLE MILK

½ TEASPOON VANILLA EXTRACT

Preheat the oven to 400°F. Line a large baking sheet with parchment paper sprayed with cooking spray.

For the wontons:

1. Stir together the banana, pecans, and brown sugar in a medium bowl. Place the egg in a small bowl. Lay the wonton wrappers out on a work surface and brush the edges lightly with egg. Place about a tablespoon of the banana mixture in the center of each wrapper. Fold the wrappers over to form half-moons or triangles and press to seal the edges.

2. Place the wontons on the prepared baking sheet and bake in the preheated oven until crisp and lightly browned, about 5 minutes. Remove from the oven and let cool on the pan while you make the caramel.

For the caramel:

Combine the butter, brown sugar, and bourbon in a small saucepan and stir over medium-high heat until the sugar is completely dissolved, about 3 minutes. Carefully add the milk and bring to a boil. Cook for about 5 minutes, until the mixture thickens. Remove from the heat and stir in the vanilla. Serve the wontons warm, drizzled with the caramel.

Baked Nectarines with Gingersnap Crumb Topping

SERVES 4

▶ CALORIES: **217**
SODIUM: **213 MILLIGRAMS**

Prep time: **5 minutes**
Cooking time: **15 minutes**

This super-simple dish combines nectarines with gingersnaps for a virtuous dessert that will satisfy your sweet tooth. Peaches make a lovely substitute.

2 NECTARINES, HALVED AND PITTED
¼ CUP GRANULATED SUGAR
¼ CUP LEMON JUICE
2 TABLESPOONS WATER
½ TEASPOON GROUND GINGER
4 GINGERSNAPS, CRUSHED

1. Preheat the oven to 425°F.

2. Place the nectarine halves in a baking dish, cut-side up.

3. In a small saucepan, combine the sugar, lemon juice, water, and ginger and bring to a simmer over medium heat. Pour the mixture over the nectarines. Sprinkle the gingersnap crumbs on top.

4. Bake in the preheated oven for about 15 minutes, until the nectarines are tender and the sauce has thickened and become syrupy. Serve warm, with a scoop of vanilla frozen yogurt if desired.

Peach-Blueberry Crisp with Coconut Topping

▶ CALORIES: **287**
  SODIUM: **6 MILLIGRAMS**

Prep time: **5 minutes**
Cooking time: **10 minutes**

Crisps are a favorite summer dessert when stone fruits and berries are at their peak. This recipe combines the two for a pretty crisp that is light and delicious. (In the fall, you might substitute apples or pears and cranberries.) A double dose of coconut makes this version unique and especially nutritious. Cooking it in individual ramekins makes both portion control and cleanup a snap. Be sure to use ramekins that are microwave- and oven-safe.

FILLING

COOKING SPRAY

2 CUPS SLICED FRESH PEACHES

1 CUP FRESH BLUEBERRIES

2 TABLESPOONS ALL-PURPOSE FLOUR

2 TABLESPOONS GRANULATED SUGAR

2 TABLESPOONS LEMON JUICE

TOPPING

¾ CUP OLD-FASHIONED ROLLED OATS

¼ CUP ALL-PURPOSE FLOUR

3 TABLESPOONS UNSWEETENED COCONUT FLAKES

2 TABLESPOONS COCONUT OIL

¼ CUP PACKED BROWN SUGAR

continued ▶

Spray four 8-ounce ramekins lightly with cooking spray.

For the filling:

In a large bowl, toss together the peaches and blueberries. Add the flour, granulated sugar, and lemon juice and toss to combine. Spoon the mixture equally among the prepared ramekins. Cover the ramekins tightly with plastic wrap and make a few small holes in each. Cook on high in the microwave for about 5 to 7 minutes, until the filling is hot and bubbling.

For the topping:

1. While the filling is cooking, preheat the broiler. Combine the oats, flour, coconut flakes, coconut oil, and brown sugar in a food processor. Pulse until the mixture is well combined.

2. Remove the ramekins from the microwave, remove and discard the plastic wrap, and place the ramekins on a baking sheet. Spoon the topping mixture over the fruit in the ramekins, making sure to cover the fruit completely.

3. Place the baking sheet with the filled ramekins in the preheated broiler and broil for 2 to 3 minutes, until the topping is nicely browned. Serve warm, topped with a scoop of vanilla ice cream or frozen yogurt, if desired.

Vanilla-Coconut Macaroons

MAKES ABOUT 30 COOKIES

▶ CALORIES: **56** (PER COOKIE)
   SODIUM: **22 MILLIGRAMS** (PER COOKIE)

Prep time: **5 minutes**
Cooking time: **15 minutes**

These simple cookies deliver big, bold coconut flavor. Not too sweet or too heavy, they're perfect for an afternoon snack or festive dessert.

2 EGG WHITES
¼ CUP MAPLE SYRUP
½ TEASPOON VANILLA EXTRACT
¼ TEASPOON SEA SALT
2 CUPS UNSWEETENED SHREDDED COCONUT

1. Preheat the oven to 350°F. Line a baking sheet with parchment paper.

2. Whisk the egg whites, maple syrup, vanilla, and salt together in a medium bowl until frothy, then stir in the coconut.

3. Scoop the cookie dough onto the prepared baking sheet using a small cookie scoop or melon baller.

4. Bake in the preheated oven until the bottoms and edges turn golden brown, about 12 to 15 minutes. Remove from the oven and let cool in the pan. Serve warm or at room temperature.

Peanut Butter and Flax Seed Cookies

MAKES ABOUT 36 COOKIES

▶ CALORIES: **89** (PER COOKIE)
SODIUM: **57 MILLIGRAMS** (PER COOKIE)

Prep time: **10 minutes**
Cooking time: **15 minutes**

Rich in omega-3 fatty acids, flax seed is thought to lower your risk of developing heart disease, cancer, stroke, and diabetes. It also adds fiber and a bit of pleasingly crunchy texture to these cookies.

½ CUP UNSALTED BUTTER, AT ROOM TEMPERATURE

¾ CUP LIGHT BROWN SUGAR

¾ CUP ALL-NATURAL, NO-SALT-ADDED PEANUT BUTTER (CREAMY OR CRUNCHY)

1 EGG

1 TEASPOON VANILLA EXTRACT

¾ CUP ALL-PURPOSE FLOUR

½ CUP WHOLE-WHEAT FLOUR

¼ CUP FLAX SEED MEAL

1 TEASPOON BAKING POWDER

1 TEASPOON BAKING SODA

1. Preheat the oven to 350°F.

2. Using an electric mixer, cream together the butter and brown sugar in a large bowl until smooth. Beat in the peanut butter, egg, and vanilla.

3. In another bowl, combine the all-purpose and whole-wheat flours, flax seed meal, baking powder, and baking soda. Add the dry ingredients to the wet ingredients and beat to mix well.

4. Drop the batter by the rounded tablespoonful onto an ungreased baking sheet and press with a fork to flatten. Bake in the preheated oven until lightly browned, about 15 minutes. Let cool on the pan for a few minutes, then transfer to a wire rack to cool completely. Serve warm or at room temperature.

The Best Oatmeal Chocolate Chip Cookies

MAKES ABOUT 30 COOKIES

▶ CALORIES: **73** (PER COOKIE)
   SODIUM: **17 MILLIGRAMS** (PER COOKIE)

Prep time: **10 minutes**
Cooking time: **15 minutes**

There's nothing quite as nice as the smell of homemade cookies baking in the oven, except perhaps that first gooey, fresh-out-of-the-oven bite. Full of chewy oats and dark chocolate, this lightened-up version of the classic cookie won't disappoint.

½ CUP ALL-PURPOSE FLOUR
½ CUP WHOLE-WHEAT FLOUR
¾ CUP OLD-FASHIONED ROLLED OATS
½ TEASPOON BAKING POWDER
⅓ TEASPOON BAKING SODA
¾ CUP LIGHT BROWN SUGAR
⅓ CUP CANOLA OIL
1 EGG
1 TEASPOON VANILLA EXTRACT
⅓ CUP SEMISWEET CHOCOLATE CHIPS

1. Preheat the oven to 350°F. Line a large baking sheet with parchment paper.

2. Combine the all-purpose and whole-wheat flours, oats, baking powder, and baking soda in a medium mixing bowl.

3. In a large mixing bowl, cream together the brown sugar and canola oil with an electric mixer. Add the egg and vanilla and beat to combine.

4. Add the dry mixture to the wet mixture and beat to combine. Stir in the chocolate chips.

5. Drop the cookie dough onto the pan by the rounded tablespoonful. Bake in the preheated oven until golden brown, about 12 to 14 minutes. Transfer the cookies to a wire rack to cool. Serve warm or at room temperature.

No-Bake Chocolate-Glazed Coconut Bars

MAKES 8 BARS

▶ CALORIES: **150** (PER BAR)
SODIUM: **4 MILLIGRAMS** (PER BAR)

Prep time: **25 minutes** (includes freezing time)
Cooking time: **2 minutes**

Besides being unbelievably delicious, coconut provides your body with MCFAs, or medium-chain fatty acids, which help lower cholesterol. These quick and easy-to-make bars contain a triple dose of coconut (meat, cream, and oil), along with good-for-you dark chocolate. In other words, they are health food that tastes like candy.

BARS

1½ CUPS UNSWEETENED SHREDDED COCONUT
¼ CUP GRANULATED SUGAR
2 TABLESPOONS COCONUT CREAM
2 TABLESPOONS COCONUT OIL
½ TEASPOON VANILLA EXTRACT

CHOCOLATE GLAZE

3 TABLESPOONS MINI SEMISWEET CHOCOLATE CHIPS
½ TABLESPOON COCONUT OIL

For the bars:

1. In a medium bowl, stir together the coconut, sugar, coconut cream, coconut oil, and vanilla until well combined. Press the mixture into an 8-by-8-inch baking pan.

2. Chill in the freezer for 15 minutes, until firm. Line a baking sheet with parchment paper.

For the chocolate glaze:

1. Line a baking sheet with parchment paper. In a microwave-safe glass measuring cup with a spout or a small microwave-safe bowl, combine the chocolate chips and coconut oil. Heat in the microwave on 50 percent power for 30 seconds. Repeat until the chocolate chips are halfway melted. Stir to melt them completely and combine the mixture well.

2. Remove the pan from the freezer and cut the mixture into 8 bars. Place the bars on the prepared baking sheet and drizzle the chocolate glaze over the top. Place the baking sheet in the freezer for about 5 minutes, until the chocolate has set. Serve immediately or store in the refrigerator for up to 3 weeks.

Chocolate Mug Cake

SERVES 1

▶ CALORIES: **295**
SODIUM: **66 MILLIGRAMS**

Prep time: **2 minutes**
Cooking time: **2 minutes**

This is the perfect snack when you are struck with a sudden and uncontrollable craving for something sweet and chocolaty. It takes less than 5 minutes to make, and the recipe is easily doubled or tripled.

3 TABLESPOON ALL-PURPOSE FLOUR
3 TABLESPOONS COCOA POWDER
2 TABLESPOONS GRANULATED SUGAR
1 TEASPOON VANILLA EXTRACT
1 EGG
PINCH OF GROUND CINNAMON

1. Stir the ingredients together in a microwave-safe mug.

2. Microwave on high for 2 minutes. Serve hot.

6-Minute Mini Chocolate Cheesecakes

MAKES 12 MINI CHEESECAKES

▶   CALORIES: **66** (PER CAKE)
     SODIUM: **48 MILLIGRAMS** (PER CAKE)

Prep time: **5 minutes**
Cooking time: **1 minute**

These little cheesecakes take only minutes to make, but they deliver plenty of creamy chocolate flavor. Serve them at your next party or anytime you want a rich and delicious treat on 6 minutes' notice.

¼ CUP SEMISWEET CHOCOLATE CHIPS
½ CUP PART-SKIM RICOTTA
12 CHOCOLATE WAFER COOKIES
6 FRESH STRAWBERRIES, SLICED

1. Place the chocolate chips in a small microwave bowl and microwave on 50 percent power in 30-second intervals until partially melted. Stir until completely melted.

2. Stir the ricotta into the melted chocolate until smooth and well combined.

3. Spoon about 1 tablespoon of the chocolate mixture onto each chocolate wafer. Top each with several strawberry slices and serve immediately.

Surprisingly Healthy Brownies

MAKES 12 BROWNIES

▶ CALORIES: **244** (PER BROWNIE)
    SODIUM: **53 MILLIGRAMS** (PER BROWNIE)

Prep time: **10 minutes**
Cooking time: **20 minutes**

Think a brownie can't be both healthy and delicious? Think again. These are rich and chocolaty. A secret ingredient keeps them moist—allowing you to use less added fat than usual—and adds protein and fiber. Believe it or not, the secret ingredient is black beans. Try baking these in a mini muffin tin for portion-controlled treats perfect for tucking into a lunchbox.

COOKING SPRAY

ONE 15-OUNCE CAN BLACK BEANS, DRAINED AND WELL RINSED

½ CUP OLD-FASHIONED ROLLED OATS

2 TABLESPOONS UNSWEETENED COCOA POWDER

¼ TEASPOON SEA SALT

½ CUP GRANULATED SUGAR

¼ CUP COCONUT OR CANOLA OIL

2 TEASPOONS VANILLA EXTRACT

½ TEASPOON BAKING POWDER

½ CUP SEMISWEET CHOCOLATE CHIPS

⅓ CUP CHOPPED NUTS, SUCH AS WALNUTS, PECANS, ALMONDS, OR HAZELNUTS (OPTIONAL)

1. Preheat the oven to 350°F. Spray an 8-by-8-inch baking pan with cooking spray.

2. Combine the beans, oats, cocoa powder, salt, sugar, oil, vanilla, and baking powder in a food processor and process until smooth. Stir in the chocolate chips and the nuts, if using.

3. Transfer the batter to the prepared baking pan and bake in the preheated oven for 16 to 18 minutes, until the edges are dry and beginning to pull away from the pan. Let cool in the pan for at least 5 minutes before cutting. Serve warm or at room temperature.

Resources

FOOD MARKETS

Sprouts Farmers Market

www.sprouts.com

A chain of specialty grocery stores that focuses on fresh foods, produce, health foods, vitamins, and supplements. There are more than 150 locations in Arizona, California, Colorado, New Mexico, Oklahoma, Texas, and Utah.

Whole Foods Market

www.wholefoodsmarket.com

A natural and organic foods supermarket chain that carries many low-sodium, sodium-free, and no-salt-added foods.

ONLINE STORES

Healthy Heart Market

www.healthyheartmarket.com

An online retailer that carries low-sodium, sodium-free, and no-salt-added foods. Here you'll find everything from low-sodium baking essentials to spices, seasoning mixes, condiments, sauces, soups, salsas, salad dressings, pickles, and snacks.
1-800-753-0310

HEALTH-RELATED WEBSITES

The DASH Diet Eating Plan

www.dashdiet.org

The website that provides information about the DASH Diet Eating Plan, or Dietary Alternatives to Stop Hypertension. The DASH Diet was developed as a way to lower high blood pressure without medication. This website provides information on the background of the diet, diet tips, and recipes.

American Heart Association

www.heart.org

The American Heart Association's website provides extensive information about heart disease, stroke, high blood pressure, and other conditions, including symptoms, risk factors, preventive measures, and treatment information.

Heart-Healthy Living

www.hearthealthyonline.com

A website that offers extensive information about heart disease, stroke, blood pressure, and cholesterol, including how to recognize symptoms of disease, how to get help, and how to reduce your risk. It also offers heart-healthy recipes, fitness advice, and information on stress management.

Mayo Clinic

www.mayoclinic.com

The Mayo Clinic's website includes information on the symptoms, causes, and treatments of high blood pressure, including medications and dietary and lifestyle changes.

National Heart, Lung, and Blood Institute

www.nhlbi.nih.gov

This website is part of the federal government's official websites for the National Institutes of Health, and it provides information on high blood pressure as well as advice for lowering blood pressure through diet and exercise.

National Institutes of Health/National Heart, Lung, and Blood Institute

www.nhlbi.nih.gov/health/public/heart/hbp/dash/new_dash.pdf

The official website of the federal government's National Institutes of Health. It offers a guide to using the DASH diet to lower your blood pressure.

WebMD

www.webmd.com

An award-winning website providing consumer health information, supportive community forums, and in-depth reference material about a vast range of health topics, including hypertension, stroke, heart disease, kidney disease, and more. It also provides information on how to follow a low-sodium diet, including meal plans and recipes.

Dr. Weil

www.drweil.com

The website of Dr. Andrew Weil, the founder of the field of integrative medicine. The site provides extensive information on dietary and lifestyle changes that may significantly reduce blood pressure and the risk of heart disease, stroke, and other diseases.

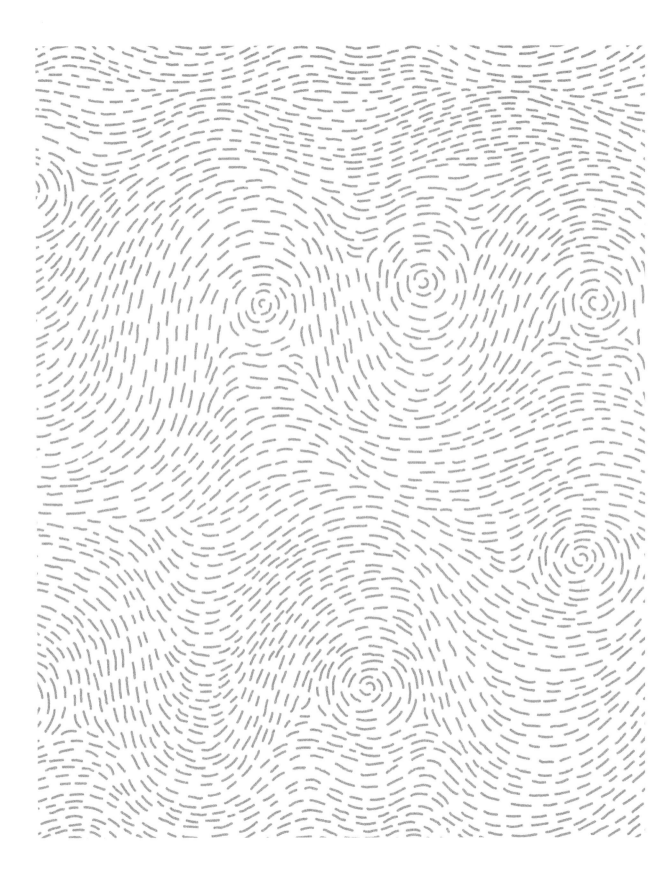

Index

Lightning Source UK Ltd.
Milton Keynes UK
UKHW051912280121
377850UK00003B/27